Lecture Notes in Medical Informatics

Vol. 1: Medical Informatics Europe 78. Proceedings 1978. Edited by J. Anderson. XI, 822 pages. 1978.

Vol. 2: D. Fenna, S. Abrahamsson, S. O. Lööw and H. Peterson, The Stockholm County Medical Information System. VI, 163 pages. 1978.

Vol. 3: Long-Term Studies on Side-Effects of Contraception – State and Planning. Symposium 1977. Edited by U. Kellhammer and K. Überla. VI, 240 pages. 1978.

Vol. 4: Clinical Trials in 'Early' Breast Cancer. Proceedings 1978. Edited by H. R. Scheurlen, G. Weckesser and I. Armbruster. VI, 283 pages. 1979.

Vol. 5: Medical Informatics Berlin 1979. Proceedings 1979. Edited by B. Barber, F. Grémy, K. Überla and G. Wagner. XXIII, 970 pages. 1979.

Vol. 6: Health Care Technology Evaluation. Proceedings, 1978. Edited by J. Goldman. VII, 118 pages. 1979.

Vol. 7: Technology and Health: Man and his World. Proceedings, 1978. Edited by G. Wagner, P. L. Reichertz and E. Masè. VI, 243 pages. 1980.

Vol. 8: Mathematical Aspects of Computerized Tomography. Proceedings 1980. Edited by F. Natterer. VIII, 309 pages. 1981.

Vol. 9: Computers and Mathematical Models in Medicine. Proceedings, 1977. Edited by D. Cardús and C. Vallbona. VIII, 315 pages. 1981.

Vol. 10: B. Fries, Applications of Operations Research to Health Care Delivery Systems. V, 107 pages. 1981.

Vol. 11: Medical Informatics Europe 81. Proceedings 1981. Edited by F. Grémy, P. Degoulet, B. Barber, and R. Salamon. XXIII, 975 pages. 1981.

Vol. 12: G. Wiederhold, Databases for Health Care. VI, 75 pages. 1981.

Vol. 13: The Computer and Blood Banking. Proceedings, 1981. Edited by J. R. Möhr and A. Kluge. X, 275 pages. 1981.

Vol. 14.: F. Wingert, Medical Informatics. X, 247 pages. 1981.

Vol. 15: Digital Image Processing in Medicine. Proceedings 1981. Edited by K. H. Höhne. VIII, 197 pages. 1981.

Vol. 16: Medical Informatics Europe 82. Proceedings, 1982. Edited by R.R. O'Moore, B. Barber, P.L. Reichertz, and F. Roger. XX, 938 pages. 1982.

Vol. 17: Biomedical Images and Computers. Proceedings, 1980. Edited by J. Sklansky and J.-C. Bisconte. VII, 332 pages. 1982.

Vol. 18: D.P. Pretschner, Engymetry and Personal Computing in Nuclear Medicine. V, 129 pages. 1982.

Vol. 19: R.L. Blum, Discovery and Representation of Causal Relationships from a Large Time-Oriented Clinical Database: The RX Project. XIX, 242 pages. 1982.

Vol. 20: S. Biefang, W. Köpcke, M.A. Schreiber, Manual for the Planning and Implementation of Therapeutic Studies. V, 100 pages. 1983.

Vol. 21: Influence of Economic Instability on Health. Proceedings, 1981. Edited by J. John, D. Schwefel, and H. Zöllner. VIII, 528 pages. 1983.

Vol. 22: Objective Medical Decision-making; Systems Approach in Acute Disease. Proceedings, 1983. Edited by J.E.W. Beneken and S.M. Lavelle. VIII, 243 pages. 1983.

Lecture Notes in Medical Informatics

Edited by P. L. Reichertz and D. A. B. Lindberg

27

Erhard Mergenthaler

Textbank Systems

Computer Science Applied in the Field of Psychoanalysis

Springer-Verlag
Berlin Heidelberg GmbH

Author

Erhard Mergenthaler
Abteilung Psychotherapie, Universität Ulm
Am Hochsträß 8, 7900 Ulm, Germany

Translator

Dr. Michael Wilson
Max-Wolf-Str. 16, 6900 Heidelberg, Germany

DOI 10.1007/978-3-662-10300-5

MyCopy version of the original edition 1985

2145/3140-543210
www.springer.com/mycopy

Preface

Psychoanalysis and information science are two disciplines that twenty years ago hardly anyone would have considered closely related with regard either to persons or subject matter. The cooperation between the two fields was made possible, on the one hand, by the development of information science from a technological discipline to a theoretically founded scientific discipline, and on the other, by the development of psychoanalysis from a hermetically closed special discipline to an open and empirical science.

This study reports the successful inclusion of information science as an instrument of research on the psychoanalytic process. This direction of work was initiated by Donald Spence and Hartvig Dahl from the Research Institute of Mental Health, New York, at the end of the 1960s. H. Thomä, H. Kächele, and their research group in Ulm must be credited with having adopted Spence's programs as early as 1974; at that time the programs even had to be implemented far away on the IBM computer at the University of Heidelberg. The efforts to expand computer-aided content analysis to a method for process research led in 1975 to the acquisition of the Hamburg program for Electronic Verbal Analysis (EVA). In the following years the author of this study revised, extended, and supplemented the EVA to create the Ulm version. This book now describes another step in the integration of information technology in fundamental research in psychoanalysis.

This study originated at the interface of psychoanalysts' and information scientists' research interests. The presentation proceeds according to the principle of trying to remain intelligible to both sides. An inevitable consequence of this principle is that technical aspects are not always discussed in the detail required by their complexity. My aim has been to describe the solution and the approaches related to it that have been attained.

My psychoanalytic competence should be considered with regard to how much psychoanalytic knowledge and understanding of complex clinical problems an information scientist can and must acquire in the course of several years of work at a psychotherapeutic instiution in order to be able to provide effective support for research in psychoanalysis.

To avoid possible misunderstandings, it should be mentioned that my reserach interests concern the exploration of complex human behavior with regard to patients and to analysts, but not an attempt to replace the therapist by a computer. I strongly caution against this trend, which is promoted by the increasing computerization of large parts of the population in the course of the current personal computer boom.

It is definitely not an everyday occurrence for a study to connect psychotherapy and information science in such a close manner. The interdisciplinary thinking it presupposes is not widespread, however it is a special trait of H. Thomä and H. Kächele, head and main assistant at the Department of Psychotherapy in Ulm. I would like to acknowledge my indebtedness to them not only for having created the institutional conditions permitting an information scientist to work at the Department, but also for permitting me to participate in all the clinical and scientific activities. If I have nonetheless been able to retain my identity as an information scientist, this is due particularly to Professor H.-J. Schneider of the Institute for Applied Information Science, Technical University of Berlin. He always made it possible for me not to lose touch with new developments and results.

I would like to thank all my colleagues at the Department of Psychotherapy for the discussions we have had and for their advice and support. My thanks go expecially to B. Drewek and E.M. Wirtz. I am also very grateful to I. Hössle and U. Kemmer for their efforts in programming, evaluating the data, and preparing the tables and graphic representations.

I would finally also like to thank M. Mühl for the diligence with which she took care of the typing, and especially for the patience she had to show in dealing with our text processor.

Ulm, im August 1985 Erhard Mergenthaler

Content

1 Characteristics and Problems of Clinical Research. The Example of Psychoanalytic Treatment.

Psychological knowledge about both healthy and ill individuals, such as can be gained under the conditions existing in the psychoanalytic situation is at the focus of clinical psychoanalytic research. According to this maxim of the "Ad Hoc Committee on Scientific Activities" of the American Psychoanalytic Association (according to KOHUT 1977, p. 118), the main object of empirical research is to obtain a scientifically examined description of the course of psychoanalytic treatment; the goals are to enable clinical theories to be tested and to let this knowledge flow back into the treatment process.

The following sections of this chapter take their point of departure in these considerations and finally lead to the concept of "text" and thus to one of the most important sources of data for psychotherapeutic activity and influence. The extent and depth of the descriptions in this chapter are based on the extent to which they can be of help in understanding the conception and the possibilities for employing the text-base management system presented in the following chapters.

1.1 The Forms for Presenting the Courses of Treatment

In the Department of Psychotherapy at the University of Ulm, where this study originated, questions are distinguished according to four levels of description (see KÄCHELE et al. 1973; KÄCHELE 1976):

1. Traditional case reports
2. Systematic descriptions
3. Scaled evaluations
4. Computer-aided text analysis.

The **traditional case study**, which FREUD took from the field of psychiatry and which remains today the most common means of description, is applied in both scientific and clinical routines (KÄCHELE 1981). Of interest to the therapist is that it can be used to describe the course of treatment in a comprehensive and integrative manner. In itself, it represents a relatively subjective method of description, the correctness of which can only be tested in discussions with other clinicians, for example in seminars on case studies. On the other hand, it is an indispensable source of information for the interpretation of the three other methods of description. The technological expense associated with this approach is exceptionally small; the therapist's protocols based on his recollection are sufficient. The regularities charaterizing the preparation of the protocols have, however, hardly been investigated (HOFFMANN and POLLER 1978; MEYER 1981).

The **systematic description** achieves a substantially higher degree of objectivity than the traditional case study. In the framework of the research on the psychoanalytic process conducted in Ulm, the systematic description is structured according to the following points of view (THOMÄ et al. 1973):

a) The patient's symptoms
b) The patient's external situation
c) Ideas from extra-analytic reference persons
d) The analytic situation from the patient's perspective
e) The analytic situation from the analyst's perspective
f) The patient's psychodynamics

These points are used by a group of clinicians not involved in the treatment process to prepare the systematic description. They work with verbatim transcripts based on taped protocols of the treatment sessions.

The purpose of **scaled evaluations** is to describe particular aspects relevant to the analytic process. A group of clinically experienced evaluators classify sessions on assessment scales according to narrowly defined constructs using taped or written excerpts of treatment sessions. Because of the large amount of time required by this method, it is restricted to small excerpts (KÄCHELE et al. 1979).

Large excerpts and whole sections of treatment protocols are examined using **computer aided text analysis**, introduced into research on the psychoanalytic process in Germany by KÄCHELE in 1976. The technological expense at this level of description is high. It requires that methods be developed even more extensively, that basic research be conducted, and that work from neighboring scientific disciplines, such as information science and linguistics, be integrated. The present study is a contribution to this task. Language is used as the primary source of data for empirical study at all four levels of examination, and to an increasing degree in the sequence the levels are listed. At the fourth level, finally, language data are used exclusively. This definitely corresponds to a characterization of psychoanalytic treatment made by FREUD, who notes in his INTRODUCTORY LECTURES that nothing else takes place in psychoanalytic treatment "than an exchange of words between the analysand and the doctor" (FREUD 1916/17, p. 43). However, he could not imagine, as he remarks a few sentences later, that the dialogue constituting psychoanalytic treatment could tolerate a third party as a listener. He taught his students that: "You cannot just be a listener in psychoanalytic treatment; you can only hear of it, and in the strictest sense of the word will only get to know psychoanalysis from hearsay" (FREUD 1916/17, p. 44). Accordingly, it is only possible for a participant to conduct research, i.e., either the analysand or the analyst. The traditional case study thus seemed for a long time to be the only viable method.

Even today psychoanalysis cannot tolerate real listeners, i.e., a third party in the treatment room. Yet the experience, some of it extending over a number of years, of researchers primarily in the United States but also in Germany demonstrates that psychoanalysis does tolerate the presence of a microphone and thus being tape recorded (WALLERSTEIN and SAMPSON 1971). The consequences, however, have hardly been clarified, as shown by RUBERG (1981) in a comprehensive survey of the literature. It is not possible for RUBERG, however, using extensive text excerpts from four psychoanalytic treatments from the ULMER TEXTBANK, to substantiate the special position often attributed to tape recordings in the literature. He shows that the patients react at least as much to other disturbing factors, such as payment for treatment or the couch. He traces the overemphasis on the influence of recordings back to the fact "that the standard conditions of the analytic setting primarily require conflict and adjustment on the part of the patient, but recordings also mean in part severe burdens for the analyst" (RUBERG 1981, p. 123). Nonetheless, the first tape recordings of treatment and their transcriptions paved the way for using the three levels of description beyond the basic level of the traditional case study.

The research approach used here has a descriptive character, as implied by the expression "level of description" used above. This approach is characterized by the point of view, following Bühler's model, that language is:

1. An expression of the patient's means of therapeutic action
2. The therapist's means of therapeutic action

A framework for interpreting the empirically acquired descriptions is gradually being developed. This especially includes models for the course of psychoanalytic treatment, and the formulation of hypotheses with regard to how models can be derived from treatment theory, which is discussed briefly in the next section.

1.2 Process Models

THOMÄ (1981) develops a process model of psychoanalytic therapy in his writings on the practice of psychoanalysis. He compares this therapy with "a continuos, temporally unlimited focal therapy with a changing focus" (THOMÄ 1981, p. 85). He begins from five premises:

1. There are regularly recurring themes in the psychoanalytic process, but there is no uniformity.
2. Psychoanalytic experience shows that it is not possible to handle several themes simultaneously, regardless of whether short or long term.
3. The psychoanalyst is an active factor in the model and exercises selective and planning functions.
4. Psychoanalytic theories are hypothetical in nature and must continuously be reexamined.
5. If the desired changes do not occur in the patient, it is necessary to change the therapeutic means.

THOMÄ does not attribute an active role to the patient, in contrast to the analyst. On the other hand, he assumes that if a focus reemerges, "the progress previously achieved retains its effect and the new handling of the focus can be undertaken as a continuation of the initial therapy" (THOMÄ 1981, p. 86). This presumes at least, however, that the patient possesses the capacity to learn, a characteristic which also makes him an active element in Thomä's model.

A process model of psychoanalytic therapy which is formally completely different has been outlined by VON ZEPPELIN (1981). It is based on MOSER et al.'s (1981) plan for a regulatory model of cognitive affective processes. While THOMÄ's conception of continuous focal therapy provides a phenomenological and global description of the psychoanalytic process, VON ZEPPELIN's description is functional and extremely differentiated, and able to fully incorporate THOMÄ's model. In her words, "New conflicts are being reactivated and forming focussed themes again and again in the analytic process. There is high redundancy in this area after a conflict has taken place ... In contrast, a new focus creates renewed uncertainty and makes new processes for seeking and gaining insights necessary" (VON ZEPPELIN 1981, p. 6). She explains the repeated thematization of one and the same focus by means of approximation models, i.e., a series of models becoming more and more exact, based on insight processes. "The cognitive work in psychoanalysis proceeds ... iteratively" (VON ZEPPELIN 1981, p. 6).

This short characterization of the focus and regulatory models introduces two types of models exemplary for the current state of research on the psychoanalytic process. The primary purpose of the following formal description of THOMÄ's focus model is to increase its transparency and to create the preconditions for a later formulation of ties to empirical research.

1.2.1 Parameters of the Focus Model

Parameters are introduced in order to establish a formal presentation of the focus model of the psychoanalytic process. They represent all the factors that influence the course of events according to the chosen perspective. The active components are the patient and the analyst. Their personal qualities and abilities determine the dynamic in the course of events, which can be described by introducing a concept of time. The focus and the conditions for its emergence are components which are passive and defined according to psychoanalytic theory. The psychoanalytic process is thus a function of these values, which can also be understood as the model's parameters. Defining them provides a closer description of the course of events.

Patient is understood as the sum of patients that can be further classified by type (e.g., types with an intact ego or a structurally disturbed ego). Patients are time dependent.

Analyst is understood as the sum of analysts. It is not yet possible to make a differentiation. Ideally, the analyst is not time dependent, but determined by the clinical theory he follows.

Time intervals are introduced for the observation of the course of events. They are fixed periods on a continuous time scale and can be defined, in accordance with real therapeutic events, as hours of treatment.

Focus serves the substantive identification of the course of events and is understood as the sum of individual foci. The focus is dependent on the patient, the analyst, and time. Examples of foci within anxiety theory are shame anxiety, castration anxiety, guilt anxiety, and separation anxiety.

Realm of Probability. There is certain probability for the appearance of each focus within psychoanalytic therapy for a given analyst-patient constellation. The probabilites can be understood as a number of inexact values, such as "certainly", "hardly", or "possibly" (fuzzy set logic; see ZADEH 1965, 1984).

Order Relationship. The individual foci do not appear in an arbitrary sequence. The order relationship provides information in the form of nonexact values about possible courses of events.

Realm of Objects. A focus is directed at one object out of the mass of available objects. Examples of objects are mother, father, and horse.

Marginal Conditions. A number of marginal conitions ensure the correct funtioning of the model. Examples are:

R1: The focus at the beginning of the psychoanalytic process is determined by the initial interaction between patient and analyst.

R2: There is an exact focus at every point in time.

1.2.2 Consequences of the Focus Model

The focus model of the psychoanalytic process discussed here is very general and certainly requires further differentiation. Before this can be done meaningfully, however, it should be confirmed idiographically in empirical studies. This confirmation in contrast to that of the regulatory model, should also be possible in practice precisely because of the slight differentiation of this model. The kinds of questions to be studied should be chosen according to the possibilities for scientific evaluation of the verbatim protocols. These points are:

1. Is it possible to demonstrate a definite sequence of time intervals in the course of psychoanalytic treatment, each with a different dominant theme, or focus? A study should also provide answers to other questions, such as: How long does the treatment of a certain focus last, both for one and for different individuals, and which range of variations does it exhibit? Does the same focus emerge several times in a course of treatment? Can different types of foci be demonstrated using these questions?

2. Can changes in the patient be registered? We can expect the answers to the following questions to be especially informative: Is a focus treated differently when it recurs? Can patient groups be defined according to the appearance of certain focal themes during treatment?

3. Is there a (possibly inexact) order relationship governing the emergence of a focus? To be more exact, do certain focal themes occur at the beginning and others at the end of psychoanalytic treatment?

This constellation of questions is exemplary in nature and by no means complete. They are appropriate, however, to form a theoretical background for the data collections and the methods described in this and the following chapters. This is also true for the following selection of hypotheses regarding the psychoanalytic process.

1.2.3 A Selection of Hypotheses

The following hypotheses can be incorporated into the focus model. They are given here as examples, since they can serve as criteria for the appropriateness of the methods to be described in later chapters. They are neither ordered nor derived from a certain system. On the contrary, they represent the (lean) yield of an information scientist's years of collecting data in routine psychoanalytic research. Until now the psychoanalytic literature has largely refrained from identifying hypotheses in the sense of preparing a paradigm for empirical research.

H1: In handling a focus from the sphere of anxiety, there is a change in the object relationship from slow to animated, from impersonal to personal, from general to specific, from inappropriate to appropriate, from abstract to concrete, and from unconscious to conscious.

H2: Unconscious guilt anxiety expresses itself as castration anxiety or castration wish.

H3: A cognitively based defensive strategy puts the object far away, and an emotionally based one is marked by cold reactions.

H4: The object is replaced while an affect is present.

H5: Toward the end of psychoanalytic treatment, themes can be worked through more rapidly. The patient is characterized by a heightened variability.

H6: The number of themes is reduced in the course of psychoanalytic treatment. This means, on the one hand, that there are an increased number of repetitions, but on the other, that this fact is associated with an increased flexibility on the part of the patient in that he can approach a theme from several perspectives. This corresponds to the patient's increased readiness to accept the therapist's perspective.

Following a distinction made by GRÖBEN und WESTMEYER (1975, pp. 108-130), we are dealing here with "unlimited universal" hypotheses that can be examined in individual cases (WESTMEYER 1979, p. 20). The essential presupposition contained in hypotheses H1, H5, and H6 is that there are individual foci. These hypotheses can be examined by utilizing "presupposition logic" (KEENAN 1972) or, to use GRÖBEN and WESTMEYER's (1975) terms, by ascertaining a "deductive confirmation", a "refutation", or the "indifference" of a hypothesis.

Correspondingly, hypothesis H2 presupposes the concept of the unconscious (LACAN 1956; LANG 1973), and H3 presupposes the existence of defense strategies and a differentiation between their cognitive and emotional bases. Hypothesis H4, finally, proceeds from the assumption that affects appear in patients during psychoanalytic treatment (MOSER 1979, 1983).

This makes it evident that empirical research on psychotherapy is really just beginning. None of the fundamental preconditions contained in the six hypotheses has been systematically studied or could be considered to be given. Solely clinical evidence speaks for their existence.

1.3 Communication Models

The reference to models of the psychoanalytic process and the identification of several hypotheses which can be used in them constitute a first and important step toward defining the goals and purpose of empirical research within the framework of a systematic approach (in contrast to clinical approaches). The following elaboration of a communication model of the psychoanalytic situation is intended to indicate possible forms of methods logical procedure which can be used completely independent of clinical point of view. The formal procedure leads from a general communication model to the communicated data and the structures of such data, to the description of language situations communication.

The multiple layers characterizing the **realm of perception** defined by a general communication model are relevant to the psychoanalytic situation in different degrees. Starting from the vocal aspect, the **textual realm** - a subunit of the realm of perception - proves to be an important, and for many questions even the appropriate, framework for empirical work. Linguistic data should thus be collected, and their structures examined.

The further development of these thoughts in this section will be based on a simple sender-receiver model, such as that described by MOLES (1971, p. 22), which incorporates elements of models from empirical social research (VON KOLLWIJK and WIEKEN-MAYSER 1974, p. 113), general linguistics (HENNIG and HUTH 1975, pp. 86-111), and the discourse analysis (HENNE and REHBOCK 1979, p. 62). Further elements will be added as required for adaptation to the psychoanalytic situation.

1.3.1 The Realm of Perception

Figure 1.1 shows the general model of communication developed in this study for the psychoanalytic situation. Its three-part structure corresponds to the partners in communication, **sender** and **receiver**, and to the **channel**. The structure and qualities of the communication channel are determined by the possibilities for sensual perception and are collectively referred to as message. Six facets result from differentiating between the message qualities. Since patient and therapist each strive to tie the communication to the person of the other, perceptions of the environment are considered to stem from a source of interference and are thus not further distinguished.

Differentiating the channel qualities permits a division of the repertoire in subsets of communicative symbols corresponding to the human capacities for perception. Not all subsets are equally powerful; for example, the ability to perceive smells is far less differentiated than that of visual perception. In addition, not every symbol can be sent

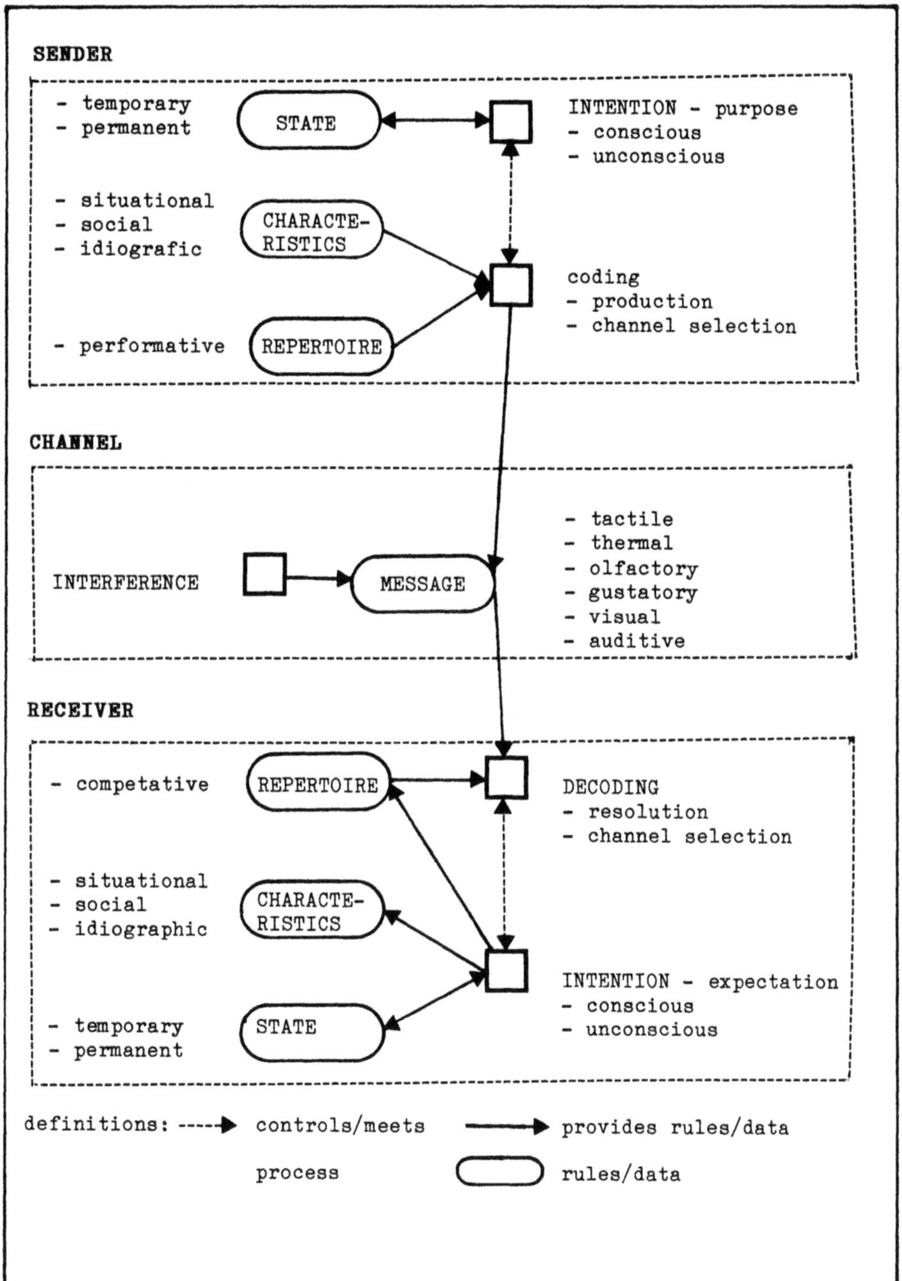

Figure 4.2 Communication model of the psychoanalytic situation

arbitrarily (intentional vs. nonintentional symbols).

The symbols have different data qualities. Some are continuous in nature, while others are discrete. For instance, the scent of a perfume can be detected for an entire hour (continuous data), while a sneeze can be over in seconds (discrete data).

An informal poll of analysts regarding the qualitative and quantitative significance of different types of perception and their symbols for the psychoanalytic situation resulted in a clear primacy of the auditive channel (see also Table 1.1). The same result has been attained in numerous scientific studies, which refer almost exclusively to the vocal field. There have also been several studies of the visual channel; examples are GOTTSCHALK's (1974) and GOTTSCHALK and ULIANA's (1977) studies of hand-mouth approximations, MAHL's (1977) exposition on body movements and acts and their role in the psychotherapeutic process, and the investigation of mimic signals in the therapy of stutterers (KRAUSE 1981; BÄNNINGER-HUBER 1984).

The **coding** is controlled by the different intentions of the sender (encoding) and the receiver (decoding): at the sender the <u>purposes</u> of the message, and at the receiver the <u>expectation</u>. The intentions can be either conscious or unconscious. A portion of the unconscious intentions become conscious during coding, leading to a correction, as is often the case with verbal parapraxes. The intentions also govern the facets of the channel to be used for the message. A denial can, for example, be expressed just visually by shaking one's head, just auditively through verbalization, or in both ways simultaneously. For the receiver this may mean that the information cannot be registered if the type of channel that is used is not the one that was expected.

The communication model presented here intentionally does not provide for data to be returned from the receiver to the sender, as described by other authors (e.g., HENNIG and HUTH 1975, p. 110), in order not to create the impression of a closed circuit. This model actually only refers to the period of time in a communicative event during which the sender/receiver roles of the participants do not change. As soon as the receiver wants to respond to the sender, the roles are switched, and the same model can be used again. The status of the participants is changed after every cycle since they have provided and received infor-

perception	**indication**	**personal examples**	**situational examples**
tactile	haptic	touch	couch cushions
	painful		
	thermal	holding hands	room temperature
olfactory	olfactory	body odor	scent of flowers
gustatory	gustatory		
visual	mimic	frowning	
	gesticulatory	nodding	
	ocular	look in the eyes	
	reflectory	jerk	
	corporal	stretch	
	habitual	fearful crouching	
	actional	open window	
	kinetic	walking back and forth	
	static		light
auditive	nasal	pant	
	oral	smack	
	anal	fart	
	ventral	growling stomach	
	manual	clap	
	instrumental		construction noise
	VOKAL*	speak	playing children
channel	**repertoire**	**sender/receiver**	**interference**

*The vocal features can be further subdivided:

channel	**repertoire**	**example**
non-verbal	paralinguistic	laugh
	conversation	interrupt
verbal	phonetic	
	lexical	
	syntax	
	voice quality	sonorous, mocking
	way of speaking	hurried
	speech control	

Table 1.1 Taxonomy of communication data

mation. In order to take this fact into account, this communication model has an additional element, the **condition**, which characterizes the changed condition of each participant.

The personal qualities and the circumstances the participants find themselves in are introduced into the model by means of situational, social, and idiosyncratic **characteristics**. These include the role as patient or therapist, everyday knowledge, and the acquired rules for using language.

1.3.2 The Text Realm

This model can be used to obtain an adequate description of psychoanalytic situation. Limitations, which at the same time amount to simplifications, result from the psychoanalytic basic rule and several very general fundamentals of treatment technique.

The **basic rule** provides the complex of intentions with a permanent component, which is experessed in the patient in his role as sender, and in the therapist in his role as receiver (see also FLADER and GRODZICKI 1978). At the same time, it sets a clear preference for the verbal form of the auditive channel. While the psychoanalytic setting does not exclude communication via the visual channel, it makes it significantly more difficult for patients to communicate in this way.

The **treatment technique** does not envisage any tactile, thermal, olfactory, or gustatory communication. Thus these channels are not used, at least not by the therapist in his role as sender and to the extent that they are under his control. This is generally also true for the patient, but it can be interrupted by behavior termed "acting in".

This model is not sensitive enough to differentiate further between, for example, intentions. The complex of intentions could comprise transference and countertransference as well as the acts of interpreting, exploring, repeating, etc.. However, the model is sufficient for our purposes, namely to gain an impression of how much the actual communication activity is subsequently reduced if psychotherapy research is limited to verbatim transcriptions of treatment sessions.

In summary, the psychoanalytic communication situation can be described as strongly associated with the auditive channel and only slightly with the visual. All other influences can be disregarded or considered as stemming from a source of interference. They only have an effect on therapy when they are additionally, as in a second step, verbalized by one of the partners in the communication.

1.4 The Limitation of the Vocal Channel

The most important goal of psychoanalytic therapy is a change in the patient's realm of experience. The therapist's most important tool in this endeavor is his use of language. The significance of talking is even increased by the psychoanalytic setting, in which face-to-face contact is limited to the first and last minutes of a session. Nonetheless, information is also being constantly exchanged between patient and therapist via all the other communication channels (see Table 1.1). It is not insignificant that every report on a session also contains a section on the patient's external appearance. Therapists often describe the patient's clothing, posture, glance, and perfume in a language full of images. LUBORSKY and SPENCE (1971, 1978) nevertheless refer to language data as the **primary data**. Yet, if the limitation to transcripts of talks - as is accepted in current research, including this study - is taken into consideration, the portion of the information contained in a communicative event which can be evaluated is reduced even further. It is therefore not amazing that some clinicians report having significant doubts as to the reliability of such data in discussions with colleagues doing empirical research on verbatim protocols. While these misgivings are definitely well founded, there are three decisive points in favor of examining verbatim transcripts.

First, there are no indications that the results from studying verbatim protocols are dependent on information that can be gained via other communication channels. The situation is rather the opposite - and this appears to be a fundamental principle in nature - in that the same information is transmitted via several channels either at the same time or with a time lag. Examples of the former are verbal denials simultaneous with head shaking, and the simultaneous appearance of a state of anxiety and of an outbreak of sweating. Other phenomena either procede or follow the verbal act. This general **principle of redundancy**, which even amounts to 66% in written German (KÜPFMÜLLER 1954, p. 270; ZEMANEK 1959, p. 58), is taken as a working hypothesis for the emprical study of verbatim protocols.

The second point concerns the affects which initially cannot be grasped in language. This limitation is not only valid for research itself, however; it is also true for the therapeutic activity, to which the affects can only be related if they are rationalized and thus verbalized by the patient or, at least, by the therapist. "The verbalization is necessary because it is only in this way that the affectively cognitive functions of analyst and analysand can be linked and adjusted to each another" (VON ZEPPELIN 1981, p. 6). Our knowledge about the process of verbalization is still very limited. MAHL (1977) presented a model (which he calls a "theoretical paradigm"; see Fig. 1.2) compatible with his own observations and those reported in the literature. Yet he himself considers important parts of it to be speculative (identified with question marks in Fig. 1.2). In this context, however, his model supports the thesis that all phenomena relevant to a psychoanalytic therapy are subject to a verbalization sooner or later, and thus can be detected as language data.

The third point concerns the desired change in the patient. Change, understood here as an expansion of the patient's realm of experience, means with regard to language an expansion of the supply of meaningful events that a patient is able to talk about. Precisely this point shows that verbatim protocols are the right point to begin studying the psychoanalytic process.

It is not possible to apply these statements to other forms of therapy or to generalize upon them to include other communication situations without further differentiating them. They are limited to the psychoanalytic talk. BODER (1940, p. 125), for example, determined in his studies on the verb-adjective quotient in drama and prose texts that differences in intonation and gesticulation can replace a considerable number of adjectives and thus remove some of the burden from the verbal channel.

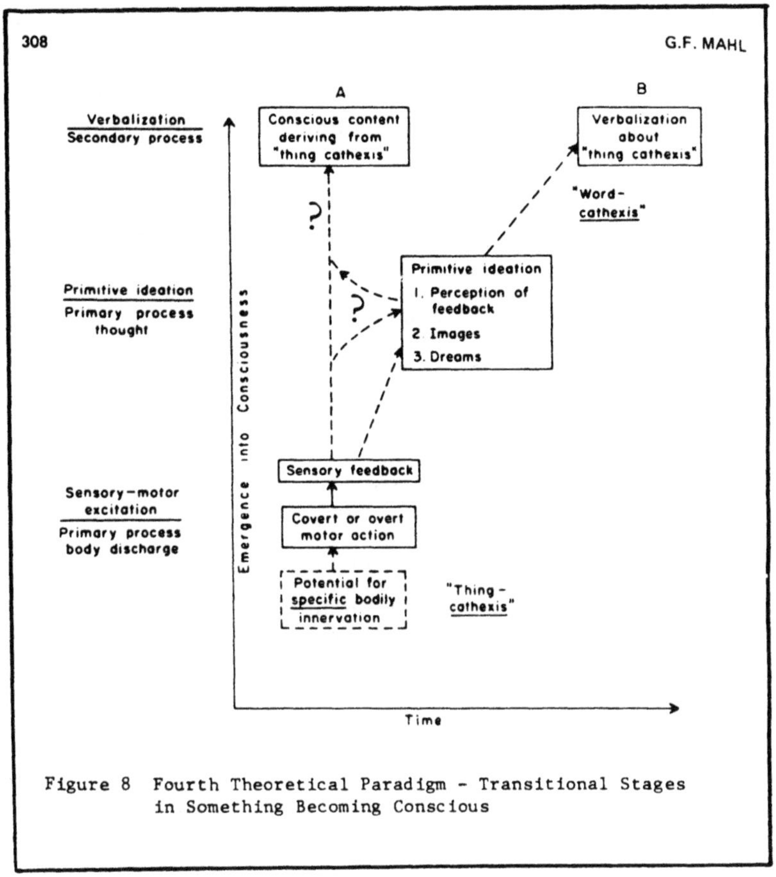

Figure 1.2 Stages in something becoming conscious

1.5 The Concept of Text Type

Talking is, in the words of HÖRMANN (1976, p. 503), an act between two people, "an act whose characteristic contours are the basis of meaning and understanding in language". Texts are the verbal precipitates of such acts. A typology of texts gives the conditions and intentions of a verbal act, and only the combination of these factors makes it possible to infer the original meaning of the act. In this section the psychoanalytic talk is described as a kind of text (see also GÖPPERT and GÖPPERT 1973, pp. 168-189). The ideas described in this regard are based on a suggestion made by SANDIG (1972) for distinguishing between types of texts by contrasting opposing features (see Table 1.2). First, however, there is a short digression on preparing the written record of a talk, the transcript, and the consequences of the transcript belonging to a particular type of text.

gesp	spoken speech
spon	spontaneous conversation
mono	monologic communication
tdia	monologic communication, dialogic text
rkon	spatial contact
akon	acoustic contact
vkon	visual contact
zkon	temporal continuity
anfa	typical beginning
ende	typical conclusion
aufb	a given speech structure
them	given topic
1per	use of the 1st person
2per	use of the 2nd person
3per	use of the 3rd person
impe	use of the imperative
temp	use of tenses
ökon	economic forms
redu	redundancy
nspr	only language forms
part	equality of partners
+	This feature is important and typical for the type of text.
-	This feature is not important or typical for the type of text.
blank	This feature is insignificant for the type of text.

Table 1.2 Features for the classification of text types following Sandig

1.5.1 Transcribed Speech

In general it is possible to distinguish two types of speech in written form: the real talk as is produced by transcribing a talk which actually took place, and the fictive talk as is written down by an author. Without making this distinction, SANDIG describes speech in its written form: "The communication is monological although the text itself is in the form of a dialogue; this is marked with the label **+tdia**" (SANDIG 1972, p. 116). Since the purpose of speech determines the rules for using the smallest language units, the functional style of a use text is given at the moment the text originates. The fictive talk thus has the label **+tdia** because it is created by the author for a potential reader and for the resulting monological communication situation. The text retains this quality even if it is then converted into spoken language, as in a radio play. In contrast, the real talk has the label **-tdia** since it was never intended for third parties. The written form of a text is irrelevant to its quality as a use text. Thus the features characterizing the talk as a type of text are invariant with regard to the text's written form or, in the opposite case, with regard to its acoustic interpretation.

The alterations which occur in a text during its transition to the written form can of course not be left out of consideration. They are based on the change in storage medium, from a real situation via tape recorder to paper. Such a change in storage medium can be connected with a more or less significant loss of information. The sources of interference may include the nature of the recording device, the quality of the transcription rules, the reliability of the persons making the transcription, the loss of the optic channel in the tape recording, and the loss of the acoustic channel in the transcription.

The description of a kind of text thus does not include information about the state of a text. It is limited to the conditions and intentions (or resulting phenomena) surrounding a text when it originates.

1.5.2 Features of the Psychoanalytic Dialogue

The psychoanalytic dialogue is a constitutive element in a form of treatment lasting several years. As a rule, the session lasts 50 minutes and takes place several times a week. The patient lies on his back on a couch, with the analyst sitting in a chair at the head of the couch. The dialogue proceeds according to the "basic rule of analysis" (FREUD 1913, p. 194), according to which the patient is supposed to yield his free associations and the analyst is supposed to listen with free-floating attentiveness (see JAPPE 1971, pp. 4ff.).

The psychoanalytic talk is a spoken dialogue: **+gesp** and **-mono**. It can be identified as spontaneous: **+spon**. Here, however, it becomes clear that while the use of forms of language not satisfying norms is a sufficient criterion to establish spontaneity, it is not a necessary criterion. The speech of some patients and therapists hardly deviates from the norms of accepted usage and must nonetheless be termed spontaneous. The observance of the basic rule of analysis itself lends the psychoanalytic talk a spontaneous character, whose consequences may include forms of language not satisfying the norms of accepted usage. In this connection, specific regularities in the divergent usage of language can be detected for individual patients and therapists. The following example is from a patient who created similar samples of speech throughout his entire 350 hours of treatment:

A: hmhm.
P: maybe also because I then somehow immediately then - somehow withdraw into draw into this role and something - what is this - I mean, I - or in the sense - in the burden or so, I have to - well, I have to take it upon myself, don't I?
A: what do you avoid by carrying the burden all by yourself;

The participants in a psychoanalytic talk have spatial contact: **+rkon**. Perceptions of everything within the room can thus become the subject of the talk and play a significant role for the course of the talk. The following excerpt of a talk shows how a visual perception can be actualized and verbalized by a patient within the framework of a defense mechanism:

A: yes. yet in the current context the point is that you accept a limitation for your husband's sake, that his erection becomes your weakness.
P: did you play football with the lamp?
A: which lamp?
P: the upright lamp, I want to see you working at your desk some time. For me work is always associated with a desk. I would like to see what peculiarities you have when you think.

In the following excerpt the personalization of the patient's stomach lets an acoustic perception be worked out as a sign. At the same time, it is an example of how a nonverbal utterance by a patient can be verbalized, thus making it transcribable.

P. now I have eaten something decent for lunch, so that my stomach won't growl again. but that doesn't keep it from making noise.
A: you let me starve.
P: starving - that reminds me that I always used to imagine that. if something didn't suit me, then I always wanted to go on a hunger strike. I always wanted to punish the others by becoming terribly thin, so that they would be worried.
A: well, being hungry also attracts attention here - you can't help hearing it.

The therapist and the patient are not in visual contact because of their particular positions. This is a significant difference to the psychotherapeutic interview, in which patient and therapist face each other. "If there is face-to-face contact, nonverbal reactions may cause the speaker to revise his opinion of the listener while talking and to organize the rest of his utterance accordingly" (HENNIG and HUTH 1975, p. 110). The label **+vkon** is used, following a suggestion made by Sandig, to indicate the presence of face-to-face contact in an interview. The asymmetric visual relationship during a psychoanalytic interview, in which the therapist can see the patient and can thus also note his body language, is given by **vkon**. Here are two examples. The first is a situation in which the therapist observes the patient and uses his observations in the interview:

A: yes, and if somebody takes a closer look, they can see that you are occupied by a lot of things and that you stare at the room.
P: and you know how to use it meaningfully.

Eliminating the patient's visual contact with the therapist is a topic in the following comment by a patient:

P: I may have never seen it right because I never really dared to look, but with you I always have the feeling that you stay snow white and cool.

Such verbalizations contradict the results of studies which claim that it is impossible to distinguish recordings of interviews using the couch from those using a chair (TAUSCH 1973, p. 43). This raises the question of the extent to which differences such as these, which are determined by the external situation, have an influence on the course of treatment. Another study mentioned by Tausch shows that there was no relationship between external situation (couch position vs. face-to-face position) and the extent of the changes in patients' constructive personality traits (TAUSCH 1973, p. 77). In view of the language differences, further studies are definitely necessary.

The psychoanalytic interview takes place within a temporal continuity: **+zkon**. While there are special language forms for beginning and ending an interview (for greetings and farewells), these forms are neither typical nor significant for the course of the interview: **anfa** and **ende**. The structure of the interviews is completely free: **-aufb**. In accordance with the basic rule, no topic is predetermined: **-them**. The interaction between therapist and patient normally occurs in the second person, and all tenses are used. In addition, the patient uses the first person much more than the therapist, and the third person about equally often. The imperative is occasionally used, but cannot be considered typical. In this connection the following bundle of labels can be used: **+1per**, **+2per**, **+3per**, and **impe**.

In the psychoanalytic interview economic forms (**+okon**) are exhibited which result from, among other things, the use of ellipses. There is a high degree of redundancy, which is closely associated with the individual participant. On the other hand, the phenomena contributing to redundancy, such as the repetition of syntagmas or portions of syntagmas, can change during the course of therapy. Redundancy is not a feature typical of the psychoanalytic interview: **redu**. In contrast, and despite the quotation from Freud mentioned above, the psychoanalytic interview is formed not only by speech and its various means: **-nspr**. The other means include paralinguistic phenomena (MAHL 1956, 1958, 1961; ZIMBARDO et al. 1963), silence (CREMERIUS 1969; BRÄHLER and ZENZ 1974; BRÄHLER 1978), and movements (DEUTSCH 1952; MAHL 1977).

Patient and therapist are not equal (**-part**) in the talk they have, as can be seen in the talk's external forms: the patient comes to the therapist, never the therapist to the patient; the patient pays for the interview; the patient lies down, while the therapist sits. The unequal positions of therapist and patient are also evident in substantive matters: the patient thinks and speaks about himself, while the therapist thinks and speaks about what the patient has said. This misrelationship is clearly experessed in the number of words they speak, the patient using about one-third more words than the therapist (KÄCHELE 1981).

Table 1.3 summarizes the features of the psychoanalytic interview. Four other types of texts are included for the sake of comparison. A complete survey of all the types of texts in the ULM TEXTBANK (currently 34 different ones) is contained in Table 2.1. As Sandig has also said, such a characterization of a text type is very rough. Refining the features would, however, make the rapid incorporation of the information about the texts which the labels provide more difficult.

	psycho-analysis	psycho-therapy	group therapy	reports	first interview
gesp	+	+	+	-	+
spon	+	+	+	-	
mono	-	-	-	+	-
tdia	-	-		-	-
rkon	+	+	+	-	+
akon	+	+	+	-	+
vkon		+	+	-	+
zkon	+	+	+	-	+
anfa					
ende			-	-	
aufb	-	-	-	-	-
them	-	-	-	+	
1per	+	+	+	+	+
2per	+	+	+	-	+
3per	+	+	+	+	+
impe				-	
temp	+	+		+	
ökon	+			-	
redu			+	-	
nspr	-	-	-	+	
part	-			-	-

Included in group therapy are Balint groups, pair therapy and family therapy.

Table 1.3 Several important types of text in the ULM TEXTBANK

1.6 The Transcription of Interviews

The rules developed for transcribing tape recordings differ significantly from what is otherwise customary (BAUSCH 1971; KLANN-DELIUS 1981). The reason for this is based on the principles, discussed in this section, for transcribing texts in a manner appropriate for psychoanalytic research.

1. The Morphologic Naturalness of the Transcripts. The graphemic presentation of word forms, the spelling of abbreviations, the form of commentaries, and the use of punctuation should be as similar as possible to the presentation and use generally accepted in written texts.

2. The Structural Naturalness of the Transcirpts. The type, paper, and appearance should be as similar as possible to what is generally accepted. The text must be clearly structured by speech markers.

The requirement that the transcripts be morphologically and structurally natural is in the interest both of the doctor and of the researcher working without the support of a computer. The doctor receives an additional copy of every transcript that he can use as a check on therapy, that is, for clinical purposes. The person doing research uses the transcripts in his studies. It is important for each of them to be able to read the transcript easily and in the customary manner. Marking inserted complete sentences, for instance, would contradict this. The reader's attentiveness would be distracted from the semantic "trail" by syntactic considerations.

3. The Transcript as an Exact Reproduction. The inevitable loss of information resulting from the transition form an acoustic to a written record of an interview should be kept as small as possible.

This requirement can in part be satisfied by extensive but normed commentaries, by the graphemic presentation of sounds and interjections which cannot be identified as speech, and by specified written forms to identify deviations from standard (nondialect) language.

4. Universality of the Transcription Rules. The rules governing trans-

cription should make it possible to create transcripts suitable for both the human and the machine user.

This requirement partially contradicts that for morphological and structural naturalness; compromises must be sought.

5. Completeness of the Transription Rules. It should be possible to prepare transcripts using only the rules intended for this purpose.

The completeness requirement means, first of all, that the transcriber should use as little of his language competence as possible, since this still cannot be described formally and varies greatly from person to person. For example, the transcription rules should not force one to think about syntactic matters, such as the insertion of complete sentences mentioned above.

6. Independence of Transcription Rules. The transcription rules should be independent of the text and of the transcriber.

This is necessary to make it possible to replace individual transcribers. This would not be possible if a transcriber creates and applies additional rules while working. In addition, the transcription rules should be applicable for all the types of text belonging to a text corpus.

7. Intellectual Elegance. The transcription rules must be easy and quick to learn. They must be limited in number.

These seven principles are ideals which cannot be achieved in practice. Furthermore, mistakes which are coincidental and may have numerous causes can occur in transcription. These include technical deficiencies in the playback machine, environmental influences such as noises disturbing the transcriber, and a transcriber's poor health. To keep these sources of mistakes to a minimum, the transcriber should be alone in a room and be able to work without being disturbed (sign: "Please do not disturb"). The playback units should be serviced regularly.

It is also possible to identify sources of systematic error. Such errors are associated primarily with the individual transcriber, and include a person's specific mistakes in hearing, preferences for certain syntactic constructions, or ideas about certain semantic sequences, because the transcriber may follow presuppositions which diverge from the original.

No systematic studies of transcription mistakes have been reported in the literature. To get an informal impression of these mistakes, however, ten applicants for a position as typist were requested to transcribe a tape. The result was ten different, in part very different texts. The following example contrasts excerpts from the text typed by four different transcribers (These text fragments mean "this morning I thought it would be good again if I could" and "it was a sexual dream. You have, then have"):

```
heut  morgen hab ich gedacht, es wär wieder gut  könnt
heute morgen hab ich gedacht,    sei wieder gut  könnt
heute morgen hab ich gedacht  es wär wieder gut, könnte
heutmorgen   hab ich gedacht     bin wieder gut, könnt

es  war ein sexueller Traum. da  haben Sie,   dann hab
es  war ein sexueller Traum.     haben Sie,   dann hab
es  war ein sexueller Traum.                  dann hab
das war ein sexueller Traum. Sie haben sich - dann hab
```

Since systematic mistakes are very difficult to detect and thus to remove, at least a few external criteria should be satisfied to keep the mistakes from becoming very consequential. Most importantly this means that a particular patient-therapist constellation be transcribed by a single typist and that no other typing interrupt a transcription. While this does not eliminate systematic mistakes, they can be taken as nearly constant and thus their influence can be disregarded when describing the course of a therapy; in contrast, the variables being studied can be expected to change in time. Given a change in typists, as is often inevitable for treatment lasting several years, it is impossible to say with certainty whether the changes which are detected can be traced back to the treatment or to the transcription. It is thus essential to identify which typist prepared a transcription if a change cannot be avoided.

Another way to increase the objectivity of the transcriptions is test listening, i.e., when someone other than the transcriber of the text checks the transcription against the tape. Figure 1.3 shows a page out of a verbatim protocol after a test listening.

TEXT: 001800 EINHEIT: 14 *NICHT KORREKTURGEHOERT* 13

*

P: was denk ich mir dann, denn ich trink an sich ja sehr gerne, allerdings nicht tagsüber, das ist eigenartig da hab ich überhaupt nicht das Verlangen danach, aber abends.

136784 T: ja, warum soll das nicht auch was Gutes haben, daß man auch einen gewissen Schutz sucht gegen allzu große Abhängigkeit, warum soll das nicht was Gutes haben

136785 P: ja aber wenn ich dann nachgebe, wer weiß wo das +hinführt da draußen liegt so ein Merkblatt, so ein Fragebogen, den jemand ausfüllen muß.

136786 T: ich meine, was ich sagen will ist, daß Sie auch da schon wieder eine Neigung haben das was Sie aufgebaut haben an Schutz gegenüber Beunruhigungen des Lebens und auch als Schutz gegen eigene, als wär das so schon auch wieder was Schlechtes. ----

136737 P: immer wieder reißt mir der Faden, das ist zum Verrücktwerden wer der Schutz den ich aufgebaut hab=

136788 t: gleich auch was Miserables, nicht wahr, daß Sie, den Schutz nur haben um ganz ganz schlimme Sachen zu vermeiden.

Figure 1.3 Excerpt of a verbatim protocol after control listening

The rules I have developed for the ULM TEXTBANK constitute an implementation of these principles. They are given in Appendix A.

1.7 The Analysis of Speech Data

A decade has elapsed since numerous verbatim protocols were used for the first time to study psychoanalytic therapy systematically. The empirical social sciences were especially instructive in the choice of instruments to be employed (see LISCH and KRIZ 1978; MERTEN 1983). The quantitative technique of content analysis, used there initially for very short texts and very simply structured categories, was to used here to discover complex structures in an extensive amount of speech material. The step to the computer was inevitable in view of the enormous task of coding (MOCHMANN 1980); just as inevitable was the increasing dissatisfaction with the results, which of course is always easy to note after the fact. The initial fascination with computers began gradually to fade. It turned out that the reality of computer applications fell far short of the expectations. It thus does not come as a surprise that in the meantime the trend has shifted to qualitative linguistic techniques, such as conversation analysis (see KALLMEYER and SCHÜTZE 1976; HENNE and REHBOCK 1979). This is reinforced by the fact that linguistics has rediscovered spoken speech as an object of research and is seeking fields of application such as psychotherapy (see LABOV and FANSHEL 1977; FLADER 1978; FLADER and WODAK-LEODOLTER 1979; FLADER et al. 1982; FLADER and KOERFER 1983).

Periods of change such as this one, on the other hand, always provide a good opportunity to take stock, and to order and document what has been achieved. At the same time we can cast an eye to neighboring disciplines, not to the social sciences this time, but rather to newer scientific fields such as computer linguistics or information science, to find approaches which may lead to solutions of the now well-known problems. Thus one question which is raised is whether the programs now available to conduct syntactic analyses of German are also capable of satisfactorily analyzing transcribed speech. And how far can the approaches to semantic analysis in information science, whether in computer information systems, research on artificial intelligence, or cognitive science, be removed from their micro-and miniworlds and be applied in a macroworld like psychoanalysis?

This study of psychotherapeutic interviews is still today one of the few scientific fields in which the central object of research is constituted by what is said by a real speaker, who is characterized only by his verbal performance. Real speech diverges significantly, however, from the competence of an ideal speaker, which is still the guiding thought of many linguists and linguistically oriented data processers. It is not unusual for phenomena, such as word and sentence parts, conspicuous syntactic constructions, the creation of unusual words, and jumps in thoughts, just to mention a few, to be called anomalies, while from a psychological perspective they belong more to the normal range of speech acts. Finally, these phenomena actually provide a significant contribution to the study of the therapeutic process.

1.8 The Taxonomy of Speech Data

The last section of this first chapter presents a brief discussion of a draft of a taxonomy of speech data. A few possibilities for applying it to the psychoanalytic interview are also given. Moreover, these ideas were decisive in the development of the plan for the textbank management system.

Starting from a semiotic view of language, which goes back to the founder of semiotics, Pierce, and to its further development by Morris, language is understood as a system of symbols whose structure is determined according to rules based on the relationship between form and content (WALTHER 1969). Accordingly, it is possible to distinguish between **formal**, **grammatic**, and **substantive** measurements. Each of these types of measurements can be further subdivided with regard to whether it can be applied to a speaker's text or to the entire speech activity in a conversation, i.e., to the dialogue. It is therefore possible to speak of **monadic** or **dyadic** values. Third and lastly, it is also possible to distinguish between these types of measurements according to the kind of data constituting them. Best known are simple frequencies of occurence, which form the basis for ratios and distributions.

It should also be noted that in the distinction made here some of the approaches for formal and grammatic measurements presume substantive knowledge either wholly or in part, such as about the denotative meaning of a word. According to the definition used here, the contrast to the substantive measurements stems from the fact that the required knowledge does not come from the field that a research task is applied to, i.e., here psychoanalysis, but from the realm of method, i.e., linguistics or information science.

The **formal measurements** can generally be determined in a simple manner. In computer-aided approaches, only the capacity to segment a sequence of symbols (letters, numbers, and special symbols) to words and punctuation is necessary. The programming task is minimal. Hardly any recoding, i.e., the entering of data, is necessary. Table 1.4 contains a selection of such formal measurements, accompanied by words indicating their applicability.

Text size (Token)	Activity
Vocabulary (Types)	
Type/Token Ratio	Efficiency
Redundancy	Simplicity vs. Complexity
Distance	Variability, Flexibility
Cluster	Fixation, Focus
Filter	Continuity
Change of speaker	Dynamic Rigidity

Table 1.4 Taxonomy of language data - Formal measures (selection)

The simplest and most elementary formal measurement is of the size of the text. KÄCHELE (1983), in a study of the verbal activity associated with size, showed that in a case of clinically satisfactory psychoanalytic treatment the interactional regulation of verbal activity led the patient to use his area of independence flexibly. However, a second patient was able to fulfill his possibilities for verbal development only slowly. O'DELL and WINDER (1975) as well use the text size as a measure of the therapist's activity in order to distinguish therapeutic techniques. They give 7% as the therapist's speech portion in analytic therapy and 31% in eclectic psychotherapy. ZIMMER and COWLES (1972), in a study of one patient who visited three therapists with different orientations, also point out significant differences. Using the same data, PEPINSKY (1979) shows that the therapist's form of activity influences the patients to act in a similar way, i.e., the speech activity of the patient conforms to that of the therapist: "a convergence of the client toward the level of talk manifested by the therapist" (PEPINSKY 1979, p. 7).

APHEK (1982) suggested investigating word systems in families as a means for research in psychotherapy. She distiguishes between two perspectives: "the first, objective, i.e., the way in which the researcher who comes from outside of the family views the communication; the second, subjective, the way in which the members of the family themselves comprehend the messages being communicated within the family" (APHEK 1982, p. 24). WODAK (1981) is pursuing a similar approach with regard to the dyadic situation.

An analysis of the frequency with which selected features of speech appear permits the identification of utterances with pathologic deviations and thus the evaluation of the presence and the stages of the course of psychotic illnesses (see PASKOVSKIJ and SREBRJANSKAJA 1971, cited according to ALEKSEEV 1984, p. 19). The multiplicity and variability of vocabulary (i.e., changes in the choice of words) attracted great interest as a formal measure in the 1940s following the introduction of the type-token ratio into psychotherapy research by Johnson and Mann. The impulse to conduct research at that time was initiated by the interest in the speech production of schizophrenics. This measure was subsequently the subject of much discussion, during which a series of weaknesses and deficiencies were pointed out. Quantitative linguistics can provide further information today, especially on frequency structures, repetition structures, cooccurence, and meaning-length relations (KÖHLER 1983), as well as more stable laws (ALTMANN 1978; ALTMANN and KIND 1982; GUITER and ARAPOV 1982; KÖHLER and ALTMANN 1983; KÖHLER 1984); however, there have not been any applications to psychotherapeutic texts.

The redundancy of a text is a measurement once adopted from information theory. SPENCE (1968) expressed some very meaningful ideas about redundancy, e.g., about psychodynamic redundancy, without being able to test them empirically. In addition, he formulted a whole series of hypotheses about the course which redundancy takes in psychoanalytic treatment. KÄCHELE and MERGENTHALER (1984) confirmed one of these hypotheses, namely that a patient's redundancy values increase in the course of treatment. The therapist's values, in contrast, remained constant.

SCHWARTZ (1980) dedicated a study to the "concreteness" of patient's utterances. She employed a list of "concrete" words, compiled by TOGLIA and BATTIG (1978), and determined their frequency in psychoanalytic material using a computer. A subsequent statistical evaluation was not able to clarify whether patients can be differentiated reliably by employing this measurement. For German, GÜNTHER and GRÖBEN (1978) developed a procedure using suffixes of abstractness, and its validity is supposed to surpass that of rating procedures. This procedure has not been applied to psychotherapy texts.

The sequence of speakers was used by BRUNNER and MERGENTHALER (1981) to detect stereotype communication patterns in families. It was possible to describe specific family systems using verbatim protocols of several consultations. BODMER (1981) and DREWEK (1984) have reported other formal characteristics of conversations with several speakers. TRAUE's (1979) suggestion for describing the interaction in two-person conversations is formal, yet includes substantive variables. MERGENTHALER (1984) provides a generalization for several speakers.

The **grammatic measures** require the researcher to have linguistic knowledge about the language being studied (e.g., the grammar of German). The programming and precoding tasks in the computer-aided procedures are considerable. Many kinds of questions can, moreover, still not be correctly processed automatically. An example is lemmatization, which can classify 50%-95% of all word forms, depending on the kind of text, to the correct lemma. The psychoanalytic interview, a form of speech with all the deficient forms (such as incomplete words and sentences) characterizing spoken and spontaneous speech, comes at the lower end of this scale. Accordingly, there are hardly any computer-aided studies of psychoanalytic texts using grammatic measures. Table

1.5 lists a selection of such measures.

Interjections		Noise
Word types		Cognitive Structure Role distributation
	Verb	Action, dynamic
	Noun	Conditions, static
	Adjective, Adverbs	Features, modal
	Pronouns	Relations
Sentences		
	Relative clause	complexity
	Yes questions	Support, confirm
	No questions	
	Incomplete sentences	
	Questions	Exploration
Phrases		
	Nominal phrases	
	Verbal phrases	
	Prepositional phrases	
Passive forms		
Tense		
	prent	
	past	
	future	
Degree of description		
	Simple	Allgeneral
	Composite	vs. Specific
Ambiguity		
	pronoun (e.g., it)	
	syntactic	
	lexical	
Diminuition/Raising		Emotion, Affect
Interjections/Text size		
	Verb/Adjective	
	Relative clause/main clause	
	Indicative/main clause	
	Phrases/Sentences	

Table 1.5 Taxonomy of language data - Grammatic measures (selection)

The distribution by word type was used by LORENZ and COBB (1954) to differentiate patients with different psychotic illnesses. To mention one result as an example, they determined that neurotics used more verbs but fewer conjunctions than the normal population used for comparison. At least in German, other variables have to be taken into account as EISENMANN (1973) demonstrated for conjunctions: "The use of particular conjunctions is determined first and foremost by locality, second by sex, third by age, and lastly by language class" (EISENMANN 1973, p. 407).

The dependence of word choice on word type and semantic class was demonstrated by BUSEMANN (1925) in investigations of children's speech. He spoke of an "active" and a "qualitative" style with regard to verbs and adjectives. He showed that these differences in style are only slightly dependent on the subject being discussed and that they rather belong to personality variables. Using a computer-aided approach to the text of a psychoanalytic interview, MERGENTHALER and KÄCHELE showed that the realization of a word from within the text may definitely depend on the subject matter, However, this microanalytic view does not exclude the possibility that, viewed at a macro level, personality-dependent variables are effective as described by BUSEMANN. The use of function words and articles by psychotics could, according to an analysis by BURNER (1984), contribute to differentiating between open and covert delusion.

The verb-adjective quotient, introduced by BODER (1940) analog to BUSEMANN's action quotients, was applied by WIRTZ and KÄCHELE (1983) to the first interviews of three different therapists. They conclude that this quotient is a differential measure of the therapist's speech style as well as of differences associated with sex and diagnosis.

Passive forms were analyzed by BEERMANN (1983) on transcripts of four psychoanalytic interviews. "Following the quantitative results, it is apparent that the passive forms can be employed in so many ways that it is impossible at this level to derive a connection proving the passive to be the category of the neurotic speech pattern" (BEERMANN 1983, p. 92). However, it can be seen in her data that it is also true that the four patients exhibit values for most of the investigated passive variables which are more similar at the end of treatment than at the beginning. It can be assumed that there are parameters for healthy speakers, especially with regard to the use of grammatic phenomena, while neurotics can deviate upwards or downwards, apparently depending on their illnesses. Psychoanalytic treatment may thus contribute to a "normalization".

The significance of personal pronouns for the structuring of object and self-relations in language has been taken up several times. Several studies undertaken on speech material from the Ulm Textbank are SCHAUMBURG (1980), CIERPKA (1982), and KRUG and KÖHLE (1982).

Deviations and changes in the endgraphy (suffix) of text word forms were utilized by WILLEE (1984) to compare texts from jargon aphetics. The results lead one to expect it to be possible to draw conclusions about the aphetic's speech intention and his residual capacity for language.

Themes	
Separation	Anxiety themes
Castration	
Guilt	
Shame	
Anxiety	
Dogmatism	Cognitive Style
Self, other	relationship
Positive, Negative	Affect balance
Primitive Concept	Cognitive Structures
Speech Acts	
Clarification	Technique
Confrontation	
Exploration	
Interpretation	
Discomfort/Relief Quotient	
Theme association	
Self + positive/utterance	
Self + negative/utterance	
Theme constancy after change in speakers	
Therapist changes the theme	Self concept

Table 1.6 Taxonomy of language data - Substantive measures (a selection)

Table 1.6 shows a selection of **substantive measures**. They presume, in addition to the knowledge mentioned above, detailed knowledge (i.e. expert knowledge) of a theory with regard to the theory's area of application. Computer-aided procedures are only able to provide approximate results and are limited to narrowly defined constructions. New approaches in information science, especially in the field of artificial intelligence, could achieve a breakthrough in such matters by establishing data bases in conjunction with a system of rules. Until now only two approaches, which, however, emphasize the rule components more strongly, have been reported in the literature (TELLER and DAHL 1981; CLIPPINGER 1974).

The most important form of the quantitative methods for substantive measurements has been content analysis. GOTTSCHALK and GLESER (1969) and GOTTSCHALK (1974) presented the scales most widely used in psychotherapy. KOCH (1984) has edited a survey of these methods, including a section by GRÜNZIG and MERGENTHALER (1984) on computer-aided approaches. LOLAS and MERGENTHALER (1982) provide a comparison between results using a computer-aided method and those from other methods.

REYNES et al. (1984) used the Regressive Imagery Dictionary (RID) to compare one patient's 10 working hours and 10 resistance hours. They obtained significant results, the working hours being determined by the primary process and the resistance hours by the secondary process. This agrees with FREUD's earlier definition of the secondary process as the one which obstructs the primary process.

A survey of further investigations using computer-aided procedures is given by KÄCHELE and MERGENTHALER (1983, 1984). The methodological discussion of these measurements is continued in Chap. 3.

2 The Textbase Management System. An Integrative Approach to Supporting Empirical Research in the Field of Psychotherapy

The Department of Psychotherapy together with the special sections for out-patients and psychoanalytic method is responsible for out-patient health care as part of the university hospital. This task is in addition to the usual **teaching and research** functions of any university institution. Precisely while fulfilling these clinical tasks, however, an enormous amount of data is accumulated; in part they are required for the clinical work itself, but they are also necessary for graduate and postgraduate education and for research. Figure 2.1 provides a general survey of the documentation and data processing in the department. At the same time, it describes the final stage of the long process of gradually integrating all the aspects involved into a overall system which is largely computer aided. Decisive is that the manual, intellectual, and automatized activities are integrated in one complex. This is also true for the archives, which are included in the overall plan independent of whether they are file cabinets or electronic storage devices. This has made it possible to pay special attention to the functional aspect, as a consequence of which it was possible to eliminate much of the redundancy that originally existed. In the meantime, the system has progressed so that each item of data is only stored once and is then, according to need, at the therapist's disposal for his clinical work, or at the disposal of the researcher working with a computer.

This chapter is especially concerned with the qualities of the **textbase management system**, or textbank system (TBS) for short, one of the three primary processes in the overview. The other two, the **data collection** and the **patient documentation system**, are described elsewhere (see KÄCHELE et al. 1983; MERGENTHALER and HÖSSLE, to be published). It is important, however, that the TBS has access to the data collection and to the information contained in the patient documentation system.

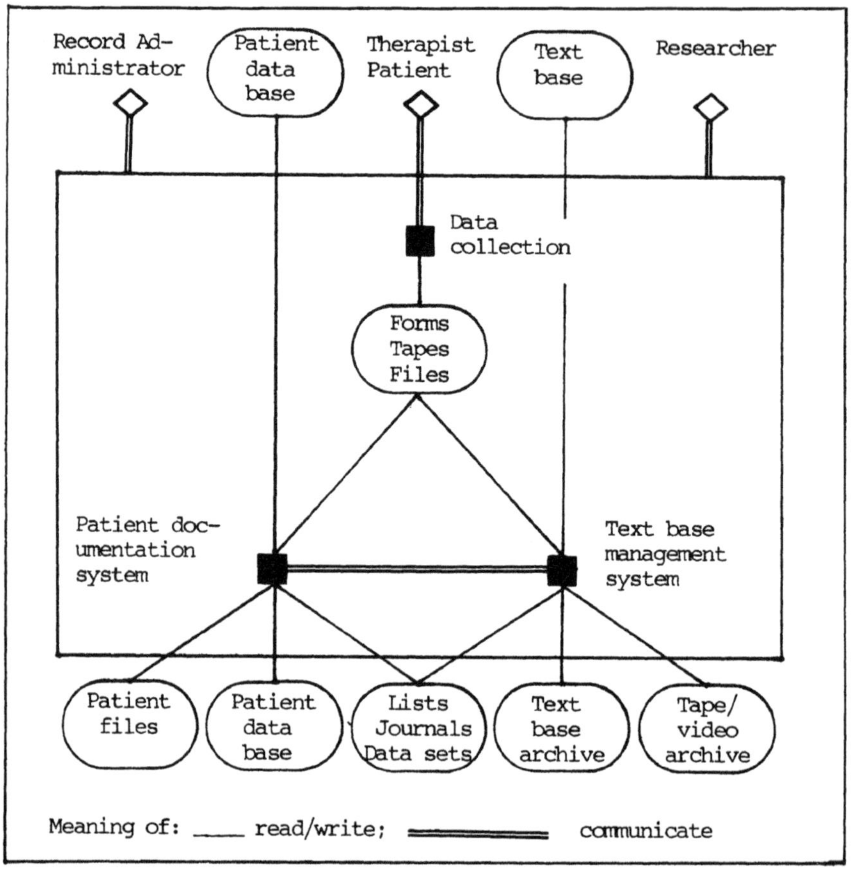

Figure 2.1 Overview of documentation and information processing at the Department for Psychotherapy

2.1 The Road to the Textbank

The founding stone of the ULM TEXTBANK was laid as early as 1968, when the first recordings of psychotherapeutic treatment were made at Ulm's Department of Psychotherapy. Initially the evaluations used normal transcriptions of the recordings; for the past 9 years, however, the texts have been transcribed in computer-readable form and evaluated with the support of comuter-aided methods. Admittedly, initially there were numerous problems in this work because the programs available at that time were not devised for such large amounts of text. The EVA system, adopted at that time from the social sciences department of the University of Hamburg, had itself only been devised to analyze headlines and newspaper advertisements (GRÜNZIG et al. 1976). The ability to apply this method without problems was only achieved after a fundamental revision of the program, which led to the version used in Ulm today.

This development also cleared the way for more advanced studies. Verbatim protocols of more psychoanalytic interviews were made, as were transcriptions of first interviews. Motivated by numerous kinds of questions, such a large store of protocols was finally accumulated that it became apparent that soon no one could maintain an overview of all the data. How could we be sure that this precious material (the transcription of each hour of treatment requires 8-35 hours, depending on the quality of the recording and the niveau of the transcription) would always be accessible, could be directly selected, and could be processed economically? The computer technology available at that time only offered the possibility to store texts as collections on external storage devices. The preparation of a body of text for a planned study using certain criteria thus required not only a good memory; extensive knowledge about computers was also required in order to assemble the desired text using the computer's language. It was thus desirable to search for solutions which could transfer this task to the computer as well, and for tools which are at the disposal of those interested in psychotherapy research and which can be controlled in a language which is both comprehensible and user friendly.

The realization of such a plan is a task of applied information science. In the general category of **computer-aided information systems** (see SCHNEIDER 1983 for the definition of this and other terms) a number of solutions can be found which are also typical of such developments. The ULM TEXTBANK project was conceived in this sense in the spring of 1979, with the goals of developing a computer-aided data system for texts and of establishing a systematic collection of texts from the psychoanalytic situation. This plan has been fulfilled step by step since January 1980 within the framework of the Special Collaborative Program 129 (Project Part B2).

2.2 Possible Applications

The TBS is a computer-aided information system that integrates three different tasks into one service:

1. Management of an unlimited number of freely definable text units.

2. Collection and management of data either describing texts or immanent in them.

3. Information about and selection of text units from the stored data.

Accordingly, the system's architecture includes modules for **handling** the texts units, for **selecting** the text units, and for managing all the information connected with the text units. The individual functions are automatized as much as possible, and the remaining manual and intellectual activities are integrated into the general system. The possible applications of the TBS can be outlined as follows: It can be used as a

1. Pure archival system for texts in different physical forms: tape recordings, video recordings, written or typed documents, computer-readable copies, and texts recorded in electronic storage devices. The services include the maintenance of different catalogues, the acquisition of new objects, the provision of data, and research.

2. Text-processing system: the transcription of tape and video recordings and transferal to electronic storage devices, the correction of electronically stored texts (called simply texts in the following) with regard to correct spelling and use of special symbols, the preparation of text for printing with the capacity to count the words and lines, the preparation of excerpts of texts according to given key words, the compilation of dictionaries for word frequency or word lists for selected texts, and the substitution of pseudonyms for the names of individuals.

3. Text analysis system: the determination of formal, grammatical, and substantive measurements of texts, the establishment of data bases.

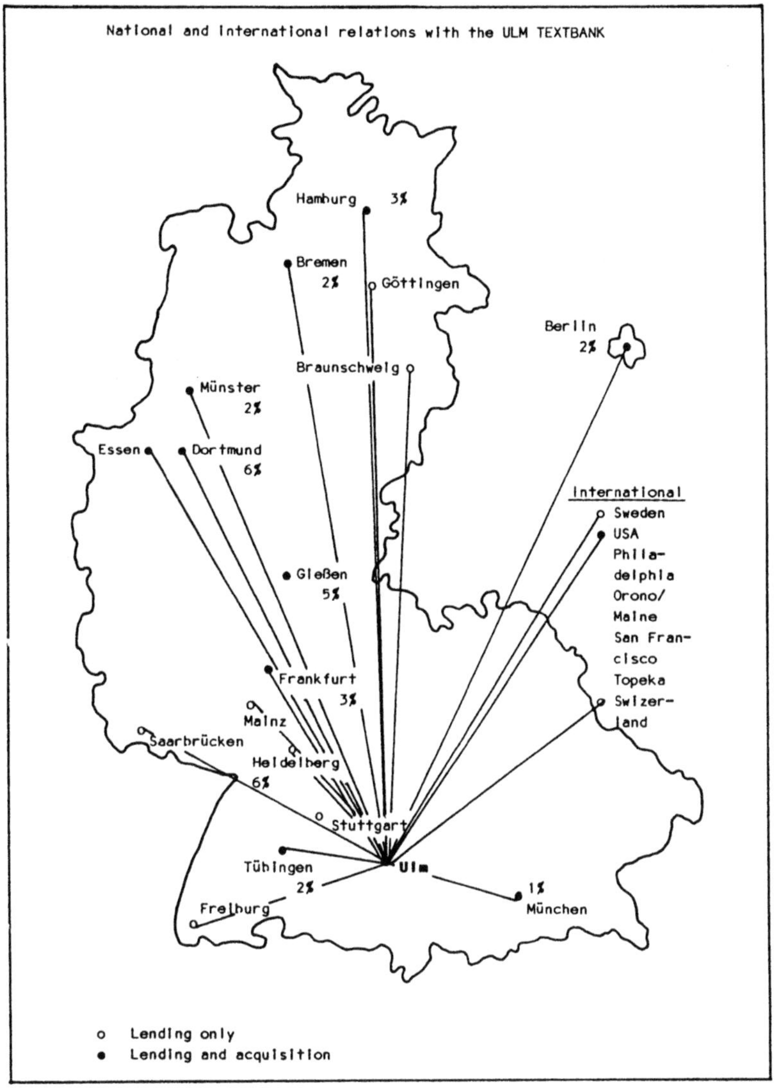

Figure 2.2 National and international relations with the ULM TEXT-BANK

Which text material is to be managed by the TBS is determined by the goals, questions, and scientific contacts of the supporting institution, in addition to the possible applications. For the Department of Psychotherapy this means first of all the desire for an empirical basis for research in the field of psychotherapy, and for teaching support in the form of demonstration material both for the education of medical students and for fulfilling clinical tasks in connection with continuing education, such as supervision using verbatim protocols (see THOMÄ and ROSENKÖTTER 1970).

As Fig. 2.2 shows, two-thirds of the material comes from Ulm. Much material was supplied, however, as a result of scientific contacts and joint research projects with institutions outside Ulm. In most cases this was tied to the right to obtain services from the TBS. While these "donators" came primarily from the narrow field of psychotherapy, the "borrowers" were almost exclusively linguists, who did not require services of the TBS other than the provision of a recording and a transcript with the number of words and lines counted.

Table 2.1 gives an informal overview of the material currently stored at the ULM TEXTBANK. The body of texts electronically stored consists of 8.2 million words. Several major points of work thus become apparent; they will be briefly discussed in the following section.

2.3 The Textbank and the Text Corpus

The optimal employment of a TBS in psychotherapy research requires that the text corpus to be administered can answer the kinds of questions which will be posed. The definition of individual text corpora as subunits of the textbank are thus especially significant. In this regard two major areas of work have crystallized at the ULM TEXTBANK; each corresponds to a different approach in research, **longitudinal section studies** and **transverse section studies.**

Longitudinal section studies concentrate on speech material from psychoanalytic treatment; their goal is the analysis of the psychoanalytic process. Because of the large number of hours that psychoanalytic treatment lasts, it is only possible to expect transcripts for a small number of different cases. Thus case studies of speech alteration during therapy are in the forefront.

The kinds of questions which go beyond the individual patient or thera-

Text type		Textbank			Tape/Video Archive		
	Number of:	P	T	S	P	T	S
1	Counseling	1	1	1			
2	Short Term Psychotherapy	4	3	14	25	8	547
3	Analytic Psychotherapy	17	11	78	8	6	782
4	Psychoanalysis	22	13	826	22	9	4557
5	Marital Psychotherapy				2*	2	17
6	Family Psychotherapy	7*	7		43		
7	Group Psychotherapy				3*	2	140
9	Group Work	4*	2		4		
11	Behaviour Psychotherapy	1	1	1	3	1	9
12	Initial Interview	300	19	308	218	20	272
13	Initial Interview Report	247	12	291			
14	Psychotherapy Case Notes	5	2	23	1	1	58
15	Psychoanalysis Case Notes	2	1	59	4	1	127
18	Balint Group Work	2*		154	5*	3	150
19	Self-experiential Group	4*	2	43			
20	Dreams	36	2	55			
22	Psychological Testing	16	1	128			
23	Catamnestic Interview	24	1	24			
24	TAT (Thematic Apperception Test)	73	6	73			
25	"Narrative"	73	6	73			
26	Genetic Counseling	29	4	29			
29	Individual Reports	-	20	20			
30	Scientific Report	-	40	40			
32	Cognitive-behavioural Psychotherapy	1	1	20			
33	Supervision	6	5	16	8	5	19
34	Psychiatric Interview	8	5	8			
	Total	882	165	2311	299	58	6678

P=Patient T=Therapist S=Session *Couple, Family, Group

Table 2.1 ULM TEXTBANK - Overview of collection end of 1984

pist and which are studied using the speech material from the first interview are the object of transverse section studies. Referring to the first interviews also means that many different patients with only one interview can be studied, which makes it possible to conduct speaker-independent speech studies of sex specificity and diagnosis, for example. Maintained separately are the text corpora required for special investigations, such as Balint group research, the study of exchanges during doctor's visits, and the study of family consultations.

The texts constituing the major points of work at the ULM TEXTBANK are being systematically increased (Table 2.2). The corpus of psychoanalysis texts now includes extensive random excerpts from four psychoanalytic cases. Individual sessions from nine other psychoanalytic therapies are also included.

The corpus of first interview texts includes several hundred different interviews and is referenced according to the **sex** of the patient or therapist and to whether the **diagnosis** is neurosis or a psychosomatic disturbance. This body of texts is supposed to be supplemented with regard to the variables sex, diagnosis, **social origin, age** (all referring to the patient), and **therapy experience** and **therapeutic approach** (referring to the therapist); this will be achieved by incorporating suitable parallel interviews.

Additionally, the general statistical characteristics of spoken speech are determined for the texts contained in the ULM TEXTBANK. A dictionary of word frequency including a concordance is updated to include every new text. General reference data are still collected for text-analytic studies; these data can be used as a baseline for specialized studies. To enable comparison of these data from the psychotherapeutic situation with data from a normal population, the ULM TEXTBANK also stores 150 interviews with members of German households; these interviews were conducted as part of a sociological study. Also for the purpose of comparison, a collection of interviews with psychotic patients at closed institutions is also available.

FIRST INTERVIEW	therapist's number	number of patient's	number of hours
	1	2	7
	11	52	55
	32	3	5
	40	3	5
	55	1	1
	81	11	11
	82	10	10
	83	10	10
	84	9	9
	94	29	29
	101	1	1
	105	40	40
	125	2	2
	126	2	2
	127	1	1
	128	1	1
	431	8	8
	432	25	25
	433	13	13
	434	11	11
	435	11	11
	436	10	10
	441	54	54
	23	309	321

PSYCHOANALYSIS	therapist's number	patient's number	number of hours
	1	1	198
		253	223
		258	1
		584	29
		645	4
		800	100
		806	2
	11	2	50
		3	102
		4	22
		252	1
		283	8
	17	582	44
	27	806	76
	49	425	18
	52	830	1
	153	6	6
	162	57	1
	163	49	2
	165	54	1
		60	1
	169	42	2
	170	64	3
	12	22	895

Table 2.2 Survey of the collection in the ULM TEXTBANK for two selected text types at the end of 1984

2.3.1 Representativeness

The primary purpose of the ULM TEXTBANK is to serve as a foundation for empirical research into the psychoanalytic process. Questions as to its representativeness are thus oriented around the goals of this kind of research. However, there are general practical limits to the theoretical consideratons which are possible in this regard. Two such limits are the large number of hours in treatment and the duration of treatment. While a sample consisting of 10 psychoanalytic cases is thus somewhat arbitrary, it permits statistical evaluations to be made and it can be realized in practice. The tape archive of 17 present and past cases of psychoanalytic treatment contains, in fact, about ten which appear to be suitable for storage in the textbank. Expressed in numbers, this means about five to ten million words of text distributed among 1000 text samples (hours). It is assumed that an hour of treatment - the psychoanalytic interview - is also a text unit.

In selecting the individual interviews to be stored in the textbank a number of points other than practical problems are important. Several of these points, in order of importance, are: the numerical balance among the different therapists, diagnostic findings which are relevant to the central subject of research (anxiety), treatment lasting 300-500 hours, and success of treatment. Other criteria for selection which would especially be relevant to statistical evaluations, such as sexual balance both among the patients and among the therapists and the patient's social origin cannot be taken into consideration due to the small number of cases to choose from. Thus it will always only be possible to call the corpus of psychoanalysis texts at Ulm representative with regard to the purpose of the research conducted there.

2.3.2 Protection of Personal Data

When entering a text into the textbank, all personal names, geographic references, and other personal characteristics are coded by means of a cryptographic procedure (RYSKA and HERDA 1980) or replaced by pseudonyms. While the texts which have thus been made anonymous (SCHLÖRER

1978) are processed on the University's computer center, the key data, i.e., all personal data, remain in the microcomputers used exclusively by the ULM TEXTBANK. This separate storage and the extensive controls on retrieval and manipulation protect the ULM TEXTBANK in large measure against misuse. The personnel working at the textbank is subject to professional discretion and was instructed as to the relevant regulations with regard to the protection of personal data. The ULM TEXTBANK is registered in the data protection list of Baden-Württemberg.

2.3.3 Availability and Costs

The services of the ULM TEXTBANK are available free of charge to scientific institutions. Charges are only made for costs resulting from labor-intensive tasks, such as the transcription of tape recordings. In return, it is expected that the texts which are added in this way can remain in the textbank and thus be accessible to other scientists.

With regard to text material lent from the textbank, it is expected that a copy of any work using this material be supplied to the ULM TEXTBANK. In this way, in addition to the actual texts an increasing amount of information on the texts but from different disciplines can be stored and made available. Further information on the conditions for utilizing is available from the ULM TEXTBANK.

2.4 The User Interface

This section is concerned with the user-TBS interface. It should give the reader a good impression of the opportunities that the system offers and thus make it possible for him to evaluate his expectations realistically. This section is not intended to provide information about operating the system or to discuss the technical data or the methodological foundation. In this regard the reader is referred to the user handbook (MERGENTHALER et al., in preparation) and to Chaps. 3 and 4 of this study. On the other hand, the **menu technique** is used in this section as a means of description, just as it is implemented in the terminals for working with TBS. A menu is understood to be a list of TBS services which are offered to the user at the terminal and permit him to mark the next step. The simultaneous use of **masks**, with which the user can insert values in prepared fields for parameterized services, makes the user largely independent of a detailed knowledge of computers. With the available hardware it is possible to employ only a rudimentary part of the **window technique**, another procedure currently enjoying increasing popularity and in which one or even several sections with additional information can be inserted into an existing terminal layout.

2.4.1 The Main Menu

After the user has identified himself to the system and proven his authorization to use the textbank by giving a password, the introductory menu shown in Fig. 2.4 is displayed on the terminal. This **main** menu makes it possible for the user to decide whether he wants to get information about the textbank or to handle tasks in the areas of text processing or text analysis. He can, in addition, obtain information about using TBS.

A **help** function is offered when a question mark is entered. The capacity to perform this function is today characteristic of an ergonomically good software product and provides the user with the permanent opportunity to determine what condition the system is in or which functions are contained in the variants offered in the menu. It is also possible to mark several variants, which are then processed sequentially from top to bottom. The user can, of course, also terminate the work with the TBS.

Once the decision has been made, the next menu is displayed to the user. Depending on the function, this selection procedure can be repeated several times until the goal has been reached. Users who often utilize the same function very soon find that wading through the menus in this manner is an inconvenience, since every step is tied to a period of waiting. In such a case the main menu, as well as several of

```
ULM TEXTBANK                                                    Main Menu
--------------------------------------------------------------------------

     _  information and research

     _  text input, edit, print, process

     _  text analysis

     _  hints for using the TBS

 _____  code for user

Please mark the desired TBS service with an x. If you insert an ?, you receive
information about the service. The individual fields are reached by means of
the TAB key. Push the RETURN key when everything has been filled in. This is
also true for the following menus.
--------------------------------------------------------------------------
     _  terminate work with the TBS
```

Figure 2.4 VDU - Layout for the main menu

the submenus, offers a field for the independent designation of a function. The user has to enter the code, listed in the user handbook, for the desired function. The reverse situation, i.e., jumping back from each submenu to the main menu, is also possible.

The manner in which the TBS functions at the user interface will be described in detail in the following section for the example of the **information and research** function. The other functions of the TBS will then only be mentioned in passing in the following sections, in order to keep the text from becoming too large. Other details can be found in the user handbook.

2.4.2 Information and Research

One of the first TBS functions that a user employs is the opportunity to get information on the materials stored in the archive and to select or do research on certain units (Fig. 2.5). Units stored by the TBS are

tape recordings, video recordings, documents, and **texts.**

```
ULM TEXTBANK                                    Information and Retrieval
--------------------------------------------------------------------------

what are you interested in?               _ tape recordings
                                          _ videos
                                          _ documents
                                          _ machine-readable texts

do you want to limit the selection?       _ yes

which information do you need?            _ basic statistics
                                          _ basic documentation
                                          _ additional choice of features

purpose of request?                       _ information at VDU
                                          _ information via printer
                                          _ borrowing the data
                                          _ defining corpus

--------------------------------------------------------------------------
_ terminate work with TBS                 _ return to main menu
```

Figure 2.5 VDU - Layout for information and retrieval

The tape and video recordings are original documents or copies of psychotherapeutic interviews. Machines are available to play or transfer the recordings.

The documents include all the text which are computer readable and are related to the units stored by the ULM TEXTBANK. Examples are written verbatim protocols, case reports (see Sect. 1.1), text findings, and scientific studies.

The texts include all electronically stored verbatim protocols and reports. If the texts are transcriptions of conversations, it is possible to subdivide the text unit into **utterances** and an aggregation of information on the **treatments.**

Selection of Units

A user generally wants to employ the information and research functions with regard to a matter of interest to him. He will thus want to name the fields according to which the units are to be selected. TBS offers a mask with descriptions of fields (Fig. 2.6) to which the user can attribute relational **opperators** and **values**. The logical OR is a relational operator connecting qualities at the same level, while the logical AND connects all qualities without or at different levels. Fields in which no value is entered are not taken into consideration. More complex questions which possibly contain further logical operators and brackets are addressed to the TBS by means of a **search language**. Furthermore, **additional fields** can be requested according to need in order to restrict the selection even further.

```
ULM TEXTBANK                                        Selection: Tape/Video
--------------------------------------------------------------------------

tape                          _  text type       _
                              _  number of hour_
                              _  date recorded   _
                              _  length          _

treatment                     _  ICD diagnosis   _

patient/client/proband        _  sex             _
                              _  age             _
                              _  education       _
                              _  position        _

therapist/interviewer         _  sex             _
                              _  age             _
                              _  experience      _

--------------------------------------------------------------------------
_  additional features?                  _  search language?
```

Figure 2.6 VDU - Layout for selection of tape and video recordings

The kind and number of fields offered by the selection mask are based on the requested units. Text size, for example, is only available for texts and can therefore not be employed as a selection criteria for tape or video recordings or documents. Figure 2.7 shows a mask for the selection of texts into which the data items have already been entered.

In this example, those utterances are to be searched from the stored psychoanalytic data that are 90 to 110 words in length. In addition, these utterances should have been made by female patients having less

```
ULM TEXTBANK                                          Selection: Text
----------------------------------------------------------------------

                          level                condition
text                        _   text type      04
                            _   text element   A
                            _   speaker        P
                            _   text size      90-110


treatment                   _   ICD diagnosis  300.0 300.2


patient/client/proband      _   sex            W
                            _   age
                            1   education      1 2
                            1   position       1


therapist/interviewer       _   sex
                            _   age
                            _   experience
```

Figure 2.7 VDU - Layout for the selection of texts

than a high school education or who work as unskilled laborers. Futhermore, only those patients are considered who have a diagnosis of anxiety neurosis or phobia.

In order to have a good overview of the selection masks, data items are not listed for the individual fields; there is rather only room to enter a code (e.g., 04 for psychoanalysis) or a symbol (e.g., for female). Users not acquainted with these codes and symbols and who do not want to refer to the user handbook, can, by means of the help function, have a window displayed which lists all the alternative data items in the TBS togheter with codes and symbols. Figure 2.8 shows the selection mask for the unit text with the window for the field for **ICD** diagnosis.

Which Information Does a User Need

By distinguishing between two forms of information, **basic statistic** and **basic documentation**, it is possible to satisfy most requests. Selection from a **supplementary list of fields** can only be of assistance with regard to detailed research or a complete documentation.

```
ULM TEXTBANK                                              Selection: Text
--------------------------------------------------------------------------

treatment                     _ ICD diagnosis ?

==========================================================================

   exhibited previously:                                     ICD diagnosis

   300.0  anxiety neurosis
   300.1  hysteric neurosis
   300.2  phobia
   300.3  compulsive neurosis
   300.4  neurotic depression
   306.2  cardiac circulatory disturbance
   309.1  long-lasting depressive reaction
   316    psychosomatic illness
   *
--------------------------------------------------------------------------
_ roll?
```

Figure 2.8 VDU - Layout for text selection with window for diagnosis

```
ULM TEXTBANK                                                    Statistics
--------------------------------------------------------------------------
number                                              min-max  mean   number

 276  text          _ text type     04                              276
                    _ text element  A                               276
                    _ speaker       P                               276
                    _ text size     90-110          94-109   104.6  276

 3    treatment     _ ICD diagnosis 300.0 300.2                     1 2

 3    patient       _ sex           W                               3
                    _ age                           23-44    32.7
                    1 education     1 2                             0 1
                    1 position      1                               2

 2    therapist     _ sex                           M               2
                    _ age                           38-60    45.3
                    _ experience                    4-22     8.7

--------------------------------------------------------------------------
_ terminate work with TBS?           _ return to main menu?
```

Figure 2.9 VDU - Layout for Textbank statistics

Basic statistics collect the important fields from all processed units and present them in tabular form. Figure 2.9 shows such a table for the example of a request given above (Fig. 2.7).

Four columns are then added to the mask that the user fills out for the request. First, at the very left is the number of ascertained units. In this case 276 utterances were found which satisfied the given conditions. These utterances come from three psychoanalytic cases and were made by three female patients. The psychoanalytic therapy was conducted by two therapists. The request is repeated in the center of the screen as it was formulated by the user. New are the Min/Max data items for numerical fields. In the example, the text size of the utterances varies between 94 and 109 words, and the patients' ages between 23 and 44. In dichotomous fields, such as the therapist's sex, the alternative which applies is listed; thus in this example there is an M since all the treatments were cunducted by male therapists. In additions, the **mean value** is given for numerical data. Accordingly, the mean length of the 276 utterances is 104.6 words, and the average age of the patients is 32.7. The fourth addition is the **number** of data items located for the fields. The number 276 appears everywhere in the example since the text units are all determined by a single data item. The situation with the ICD diagnosis is different, with the items 300.0 and 300.2 each appearing once. Because schooling and work are in an OR link (each at the level 1), it is completely plausible that 2, for schooling, was the only data item found, the other two patients being qualified higher than 1 for work.

Thus basic documentation presents the most important fields in tabular form for each unit located. The user can delve further into the material by viewing information at the terminal or in the printed lists. Figure 2.10 shows the displayed contents for the request discussed above (Fig. 2.7).

For the basic documentation the terminal displays the missing data items for each utterance as requested by the user. This example shows the utterance with the internal TBS identification number 001207 as the fourth of the 276 located items. The length of this utterance is 98 words, the diagnosis is anxiety neurosis, the patient's age is 31, she has a grammar school education and a medium position at work. Since these two fields were linked with an OR in the request, the identification is correct because it was made via the amount of school education. The therapist in this treatment is male and 60 years old, and has 22 years of professional experience. By means of the menu line the user can then either leaf (i.e., request further information to this utterance), request the next utterance, or terminate the function and return to the selection distribution.

```
ULM TEXTBANK                                                  Documentation
----------------------------------------------------------------------------

text                      _ text type      04                  ID: 001207
                          _ text element   A
                          _ speaker        P
                          _ text size      98

treatment                 _ ICD diagnosis  300.0

patient/client/proband    _ sex            W
                          _ age            31
                          1 education      2
                          1 position       2

therapeut/interviewer     _ sex            M
                          _ age            60
                          _ experience     22

----------------------------------------------------------------------------
_ roll                    _ continue?    _ terminate?          No. 4 of 276
```

Figure 2.10 VDU - Layout for the documentation of data

Supplementary fields are available for a series of units and can also be incorporated in the lists when desired. To do this, the user can name all the fields of interest to him in another interactive step on a mask. These are then incorporated into the basic statistics and the basic documentation as needed. The user also still has the possibility to select the variant ALL instead of individual fields; the user then receives the complete statistics or documentation.

What Is the Purpose of the Request?

The motivations of TBS users may be very different. While one person merely wants to get an **informal** impression at a terminal, another requires an extensive **documentation** in printed form to work with independent of the computer. Still another had already been informed and now wants to **borrow** the units he selected. Finally, a fourth person would like to define a **corpus** in order to be able to evaluate it in its entirety.

No further explanation is needed here about the information services supplied at the display screen or by the printer. Borrowing selected units, however, is connected with several special features. The TBS must first verify that a copy of the conditions on borrowing has been signed by the user. Otherwise he must be requested to comply with this administrative act, which is manditory for reasons of data privacy. The TBS then stores the borrower's wish and fulfills it as soon as the signature has been submitted and entered into the system by the TBS administrator. Then a work schedule is compiled for the preparation of copies of tapes, for the availability of documents, or for the printing of texts, depending on the kind of unit which was requested.

2.4.3 Text Input, Editing, and Printing

The TBS functions summarized here include all the tasks that can, in short, be referred to by the concept of **text processing**. They are used primarily by the personnel entrusted with the organization and maintenance of the textbank in the TBS.

Text Input

The TBS provides for four methods of text input: Via a **data display terminal**, via **machine-readable documents**, via **electronic storage media**, and via **long-distance transmission**. Thus in practice there is a route open to anyone who is interested in inputting texts into the textbank.

In the future the standardized route will be to input data via a data display terminal, while the machine-readable document will only be employed in exceptional cases, such as in a doctor's office not equipped for data processing. Electronic storage media will be the medium of choice for exchanges between international contacts. Long-distance data transmission will achieve, on the other hand, special significance in the domestic field. Especially noteworthy will be the connection of the ULM TEXTBANK onto the German Research Network.

Text Editing

When texts are initially input into the textbank, they will be subject to a thorough analysis. Special attention will be paid to the correction of typing and transcription mistakes. In a three-stage procedure, intellectual and computer-aided steps are integrated into a homogeneous system to **ensure quality.** One aspect of this procedure is the distribution of pseudonyms for personal and geographic names in order to guarantee true anonymity of the data. The quality control starts from an uncorrected text, which then passes through text correction and text control, with one final correction stage before the procedure ends with the input of the examined and anonymous text.

First to the text correction procedure: After a text has been input into the TBS, it is first compared with the basic vocabulary of the ULM TEXTBANK. Then the text is printed with all the words not contained in the basic vocabulary appearing in red. These red word forms are names, typing mistakes, and words not yet contained in the basic vocabulary. In the subsequent intellectual, but computeraided, step, all the red words are displayed singly on the processor's display screen, and his instructions for corrections are entered and carried out. For incorrectly written words this means the input of the correct spelling, for names a note as to whether a pseudonym should be entered, and for the word forms new to the TBS the suggestion that they be incorporated into the basic vocabulary. Thus in questionable cases the "red print" can be profitably employed to aid in a decision based on the context. In addition, the system may have further questions, such as to a new word's type. Furthermore, all user entries are stored in a small memory so that red words occurring several times in a text are not asked more than once, but are processed according to the first correction instruction.

The procedure described here is oriented toward the pragmatic goal of being able to correct texts with as little effort as possible. Yet it cannot guarantee that a text is free of mistakes, because a simple check against a vocabulary does not mean that all typing mistakes will be recognized. To name an example, by confusing a "y" and a "b" "joy" becomes "job" and both words may be in the basic vocabulary. Procedures capable of recognizing such mistakes are still in the experimental stage and thus cannot be employed in a production system at this time. In its place another quality control step, the text control, is used. This step must always be used during the transcription process anyway (see Sect. 1.6 and Appendix A).

The text control starts from an edited printout of the text, containing all the corrections made in the first step. The printout can now, in another intellectual stage, be either proofread or - for transcriptions - checked against the tape. All alterations are first made by hand on the printout and then, using the computer again, on the stored text itself. The red print procedure is then repeated, producing the final version of the text which can be filed. The number of typing mistakes still in the text is less than 1 % according to studies of samples taken from the ULM TEXTBANK.

Text Printing

A large portion of the TBS functions are associated with the printing of texts. For this reason special value was placed on a flexible print program from the inception of the TBS. The most important variants which the user can choose from are:

- Structuring of conversational texts to utterances
- Flexible identification of the speaker
- Optional line count
- Optional word count
- Emphasis or attribution of individual words
- Different DIN formats

The print function also includes the preparation of KWIC lists, permitting the context to be printed for selected words. As an example of such a list see figure 2.11.

2.4.4 Text Analysis

This TBS function provides the user with the opportunity to utilize a wealth of different procedures to analyze language data (see also Sect. 1.8). The number of analysis procedures available is open and can be increased to correspond to the developments in different research areas. The integration of a complete bibliography on computer applications in psychotherapy into the ULM TEXTBANK is foreseen; the user will thus be able to familiarize himself with a subject matter when selecting a procedure. Experience has shown that such support services are especially helpful precisely for psychologists and doctors working primarily in psychotherapy research because they generally understand little about computer-aided text analysis procedures as a result of the prevailing patterns of education.

Another advantage is that the TBS knows which texts have been analyzed with which procedures. In the course of time a wide spectrum of results on one set of data will thus become available.

29	h= das ist das eine und dann=	**brauch**	ich= mindestens jede zw
35	mehr mit denen mache und die	**muß**	ich dann immer zu mir hole
38	u mir holen und und +hm ich	**muß+**	mich vorbereiten. also da
73	t es, ja. eh drei Stunden eh	**nötig**	sind um= wirklich auch d
75	ich auch die Themen ja damit	**muß**	ich / / / durchzuarbeiten
83	o mit Ihnen vorher besprechen	**sollen,**	früher. ich mein ich h
99	11 gemacht, (lacht etwas) und	**muß**	das alles selber bezahlen=
143	nd und eh da war meine Mutter	**schuld**	aber ich muß das eben d
143	meine Mutter schuld aber ich	**muß**	das eben doch alles zahlen
145	d eh dann haben sie mir keine	**richtigen**	Reifen montiert und
147	ßlich, weiter das ist keine	**richtigen**	auf eh also ich hab
148	stellt Gürtelreifen, und mein	**Gott**	jetzt reden wir vom Auto.
214	h früher mit Ihnen besprechen	**sollen,**	vor den Ferien, also d
227	so ich eh eh= das Finanzielle	**sollte**	meines Erachtens da nic
234	ie nicht ganz glaube ich eh=	**berechtigt**	ist. eh= ja. ja.
280	e, aber das mit den Mädchen	**muß**	also drin sein weil= das i
282	jetzt als Zehnte und und die	**muß**	ich ein bißchen hm nich
309	nd vor dem Auto hab ich jetzt	**regelrecht**	Angst= hm eh in j
329	h hätte eigentlich eher sagen	**sollen,**	ich würd nicht glauben
388	entlich auch es besser Wissen	**müßte**	von berufswegen. ja, in
389	ist der Beruf nicht so ganz	**+richtig**	gewesen ja, ja, hm+
460	das= buchstäbliche schlechte	**Gewissen**	von mir= eh bei dem e
473	tuation wo man ein schlechtes	**Gewissen**	haben könnte obwohl w
475	agt hab, die Cousine, eh sie	**sollen**	sich nicht wundern das=
477	as das war eigentlich nichts=	**Negatives.**	aber ich hätte doch
481	ich getan haben könnte oder	**sollte**	und -- meine Mutter sie
484	fertig, wenn es jemand stört	**soll**	er mir´s sagen.´ -- und d
489	ze jeder ist für sein Gesicht	**verantwortlich**	und man kann ni
493	ist wenn irgendjemand eh was	**Negatives**	hat oder oder denkt
520	ch dann= unsicher und und eh	**verrückt,**	wenn irgendsowas auf
527	tte auf.´ - und das geht dann	**recht**	zügig und fertig. aber i
538	hen. genau. hm und und= er	**sollte**	eigentlich dann zu den
544	und, ich hatte mich wirklich	**korrekt**	verhalten, und dachte
546	nweisen daß man jetzt nicht	**verrückt**	spielen soll´ oder so
547	jetzt nicht verrückt spielen	**soll´**	oder so. hm und= - ich
550	enau wußte ich hatte es nicht	**falsch**	gemacht. ja, und dann h
555	en und, mich würde es einfach	**verrückt**	machen. und= er war n
565	h mal stellvertretend rot und	**mußte**	dann abwarten, bis sich
586	immer= irgendwie sich in die	**Rolle=**	von den andern versetzt
602	ir zugewiesen hat oder seine=	**Rollen**	vollends durchgeführt o
606	ht bloß so= stellvertretendes	**Schuldgefühl**	sondern wirklich=
611	ht, - was da alles die letzte	**Rolle**	spielte. ---- ach ja, es
613	en daß man mal ein schlechtes	**Gewissen**	hatte wenn man was sa
618	wußte daß daß da nichts hm= -	**Inkorrektes**	dabei war und, und
620	schlecht behandelt oder nicht	**korrekt**	behandelt zu haben, -
622	irklich ja keine Lust da= der	**Sündenbock**	zu sein und= ---- e
625	es könnte doch irgend etwas	**falsch**	aufgefaßt werden. - auc
625	faßt werden. - auch was nicht	**falsch**	aufzufassen sei weil ic
654	s mal einen Streit - oder man	**mußte**	sich einfach entschuldig
658	irgend so ein pauschales, eh	**Schuldgefühl**	vermitteln und un
680	Augen nicht mehr, die an sich	**recht**	gut sehen. hm denn ic
695	und ich glaub es war nur so	**Theologie**	und Sport und so wei

Figure 2.11 Sample Key-Word-In-Context Listing (KWIC)

3 The Textbase Management System: A Method Base for Text Editing and Analysis

The third chapter of this study is concerned with the TBS in its capacity as a method base for processing the linguistic data contained in psychotherapeutic texts. After a short introductory section, some basic concepts will be defined; this should aid in the description of the methodical steps in the subsequent sections. The third section deals with single algorithms, such as are required for the restructuring, editing, and reproduction of texts. Then the problems associated with spoken speech and sampling size will be discussed briefly. The last section of this chapter is dedicated to one important aspect of the TBS, namely, to the integrated word data base.

3.1 Introduction

The study of natural language texts from practical points of view is of special significance in many areas of research. Researchers always find that using the methods from content analysis involves great expense and is laborious. It is thus understandable that many people placed great hopes in computers as language processors as soon as it became possible to program computers to read and write, and not merely to compute. Yet after the first one-to-one translations from English into German produced such miserable results, to mention a very unfavorable example, these hopes disappeared quickly. It became apparent that linguistics did not have any theories to offer which could have been applied fruitfully in information science. Thus speech statistics and word field theory remained two of the most important points of departure for machine analysis of language. Significant developments and progress were made in this regard in the period 1965-1970.

The system General Inquirer (STONE et al. 1966) was developed as a prototype for computer-aided content analysis and achieved a position of special importance in the social sciences. Regarding the psychotherapeutic scope of application, LAFFAL's (1968) "total content analysis" can be mentioned. Although the methodological foundations were distinctly different in the work of STONE et al. and LAFFAL, the computerized text analysis process followed the same schema for both. The preliminary task is the compilation of a glossary or dictionary, often consisting of a collection of several thousand word forms which are assigned to different categories themselves constitute a system including either the facets to a special topic or the aspects of a more general complex of topics. The vocabulary of a dictionary can be derived either inductively from a text or deductively from more general constructs whose consequences can be detected in the choice of categories. The computer's task is to examine a text word for word and to compare it to the dictionary. If a word form is found, the number of entries counted for the corresponding category is increased by one. The resulting frequency distribution can also be relativized at the beginning of the text for the purposes of comparison. Depending on the system, this fundamental algorithm can be modified into a more or less elaborate form by the introduction of additional rules. STONE et al., for example, attempt in this manner to resolve the ambiguity of many word forms (in German more than 60%) by referring to the context. This level of development characterizes computer-aided content analysis even today, including the systems commonly used where German is spoken (Textpack, LDVLIB, and EVA). It can be considered an independent method that, however, has never gone beyond the scope of its application in the empirical social sciences.

Computer scientists and linguists went through another wave of hope during the reception of CHOMSKY's (1965) syntax theory. The former were enthusiastic with the rules provided by CHOMSKY's generative grammar, which seemed to be created just for the computer; the latter were happy finally to have a grip on language and to be able to test their theories empirically (see FRIEDMAN 1969, 1971, 1973). How far their efforts have brought them is described in informal terms by the heading of a newspaper article written by a linguist: Big Man - What Now? (WEINRICH 1975). The generative approach is marred by two faults. First, it is a theory of competence which applies only to an ideal speaker, who does not exist in reality. Second, despite several important attempts (see KATZ and FODOR 1964), no adequate theory of semantics has been developed to supplement the syntax theory. It is thus not surprising that no program has been developed out of this approach which can be applied in practice to analyze texts.

Yet "meaning" and "understanding" are words which today are no longer foreign with regard to computers (HÖRMANN 1976). While content analysts primarily concentrated on the implementation of their modest methods and CHOMSKY grammaticians became increasingly entangled in their rules, scientists from other fields have attempted to use comuters in very pragmatic ways to reproduce the smallest areas of human intelligence. Initially language did not play any role in these approaches. This situation was decisively altered, however, by WINOGRAD's SHRDLU (WINOGRAD 1972) - a robot who demonstrated all kinds of intelligence in a microworld of cubes. The field today known as cognitive science developed; its primary object of study is computers' understanding of language (SCHANK 1980). Studies in this field find applications, for example, in the preparation of abridged versions of stories or articles, the organization of data bases, and answering natural language requests in information systems. While these tasks can today be solved surprisingly well, they are restricted to narrowly limited areas of discourse and thus so far to fields other than psychotherapy research.

3.2 Basic Concepts

The following list of basic concepts is included as an aid to the person trying to use the services provided by the TBS. Such a definition of terms has proven itself useful in the past since the everyday meaning of some of the terms diverges from the special meaning in the field of computers.

Word Form (1)

A word form is every word said by a speaker of a natural language. In the written presentation of speech, word form refers to a sequence of letters bordered by spaces or special symbols.

Examples of word forms are the words: I, gone, houses, humm.

Comment: In general linguistics this definition corresponds to a series of graphemes. There a word form can consist of several, not necessarily sequential, series of graphemes; for example, "will have eaten" is a word form consisting of three groups of graphems. In a sentence this word form may be interrupted by other graphemic groups: "Tomorrow I will only have eaten lunch or had a snack." The recognition of such word forms with the aid of algorithmic procedures requires extensive syntactic and semantic analyses of the context. In many cases, the end of the sentence does not sufficiently limit the context, so that the entire text may possibly have to be referred to.

Basic Form (2)

Basic forms are all uninflected word forms. For verbs this is the infinitive, for nouns the nominative singular, and for adjectives the positive. Thus for one basic form there may be several word forms.
Examples of basic forms are the words: I, go, house, humm.

Comment: Corresponding to the definition of word form used here, the concept of basic form also refers to a series of graphemes: "will have eaten" thus refers to the three basic forms "will", "have", and "eat".

Complete Form (3)

A complete form is an inflexted word form, and for every complete form there is a basic form.
Examples of complete forms are: me, went, houses.

Word Lists (4)

A word list is a finite quantity of different word forms.

Lemma (5)

A lemma is a quantity of word forms grouped together because of their agreement with regard to given qualities.
Examples of lemmata are the word entries in a dictionary.

Comment: General linguistics distinguishes between syntagmatic, paradigmatic, and structural qualities. A second condition is usually that a lemma only includes word forms of one word kind and with one root.

Lemma Dictionary (6)

A lemma dictionary is a structured quantity of lemmata. Every single lemma is determined by a congruence of the word kind and the meaning of all the word forms belonging to it. The corresponding basic form is used as the lemma name.
Examples for the entries in a lemma dictionary are the lemmata:

residence = (residence, residences)

and

reside = (reside, resided, residing, resides)

Word Kind (7)

A word kind is the role a word form fulfills in speech or in sentence structure (see ERBEN 1968, pp. 38ff.). The following word kinds are distinguished:

- Verbs
- Nouns
- Adjectives
- Pronouns
- Prepositions and conjunctions
- Adverbs and predicate adjectives

Verbs amount to about a fourth of the entire vocabulary and are the main means of statements (rheme) describing action or a state of being. Nouns constitute more than two-thirds of the entire vocabulary and serve to name the significant aspects (themes) surrounding an action or determining a state of being. Adjectives constitute about a sixth of the entire vocabulary and serve to characterize a given act or state of being and the significant aspects involved in it. The pronouns, prepositions, conjunctions, and adverbs together amount to about a tenth of the entire vocabulary; their function is to supplement the three main word kinds by enabling references, relationships, connections, and modal and emotional expressions to be made.

Comment: This functionally and syntactically oriented definition of word kind takes especially the pragmatic goals of the desired text analysis into account.

Word Form Index (8)

A word form index is a structured list of all the word forms appearing in a text. The frequency of a word's appearance is also recorded for each word form.

Basic Form Index (9)

A basic form index is a list of all the word forms appearing in a text which have been traced back to their basic forms. The frequency of a word's appearance is recorded for each basic form.

Comment: Word and basic form indexes constitute the basis of frequency dictionaries. A comprehensive description is given by ALEKSEEV (1984).

Category (10)

A category refers to the names of open quantities of word forms grouped under the same substantive point of view. For example, all word forms which refer to sensual perceptions could be grouped under the category "sense".

System of Categories (11)

A system of categories is a quantity of categories which is self-contained according to substantive points of view. For instance, the system of categories Anxiety Themes includes the categories Shame, Castration, Guilt, and Separation.

Vocabulary (12)

Vocabulary refers to an index of word forms or of basic forms if the distinction between complete form and basic form is not relevant.

Dictionary (13)

A dictionary is a finite quantity of ordered pairs. Every pair consists of a word form and a category. For example, given the word list:

W = (cut_off, cutting_off, soon, knife, judgement, judgements)

and

C = (Shame, Castration, Guilt, Separation)

a dictionary which corresponds to the definition given here might look as follows:

D = (cut_off, Castration; cutting_off, Castration; cut_off, Separation; cutting_off, Separation; knife, Castration; knife, Guilt; judgement, Guilt; judgements, Guilt)

Such a dictionary can also be understood as a relation between word list W and the system of categories C, and thus as a subquantity of the Cartesian product W x C. To obtain the desired subquantity in the form of a dictionary, secondary conditions can be agreed upon, the most common of which are:

C1: For every pair of elements in subquantity D, the meaning of the given word forms should agree with the definition of the category associated with them.

This excludes the "meaningless" pairs of elements from the complete Cartesian product. Since this condition was applied to the above-mentioned example, the pair of elements (soon, Guilt) is not given as an item in D.

C2: Each word form in the word list W may appear in only one pair of elements in the subquantity D.

This agreement prevents multiple classifications. If C2 is applied to the above-mentioned example, a decision must be made as to the category under which the word forms "cut_off", "cutting_off", and "knife" will be included in the dictionary. Consequently the following dictionary might result:

D = (cut_off, Castration; cutting_off, Castration; knife, Castration; judgement, Guilt; judgements, Guilt)

C3: Excluding inflected word forms makes dictionaries smaller and easier to use. Applying C3 to the example produces the following dictionary:

D = (cut_off, Castration; knife, Castration; judgement, Guilt)

Standard Dictionary (14)

Standard dictionaries are dictionaries satisfying the secondary conditions C1, C2, and C3.

Text (15)

A text is a structured quantity of word forms, punctuation marks, and commentaries. Symbols identifying speakers do not belong to the text itself, but label a text. A text can be organized hierarchically. The following levels are distinguished in therapeutic conversations:

- Word form
- Utterance
- Session (hour)
- Sequence of sessions (treatment)

Standard text (16)

A standard text is a text whose word forms have been traced back to basic forms. A standard text thus does not contain any complete forms, but its structure (and therefore the sequence of the word forms) is retained.

Type (17)
All the different word forms appearing in a text or a word list are called types.

Token (18)
All the word forms appearing in a text or word list are called tokens. The number of tokens always corresponds to the text size.

Corpus (19)
A corpus is a quantity of text which is grouped together under one general point of view. For example, the ULM TEXTBANK comprises a corpus which contains texts form the psychotherapeutic situation. Subcorpora can also be defined; for instance, the collection of first interviews selected on the basis of the patient's sex and age constitutes a limited subcorpus.

3.3 Processing

The algorithmic processing of texts with the methods available within the framework of the ULM TEXTBANK is possible according to two points of view. First, a text can be viewed as a quantity of word forms and processed according to a quantity-oriented procedure. The other view follows the sequential structure of word forms in the text; such procedures are called structure oriented.

3.3.1 Quantity-Oriented Processing

Preparation of a Word Form Index (A1)
Word forms, together with frequency of occurrence, which appear in a text are determined, sorted either alphabetically or according to fre-

quency of occurence, and made available as a file or a printout.

Preparation of a Basic Form Index (A2)

A basic form index can be prepared from either a text or a previously prepared word form index. All the complete forms which occur are traced back to their basic forms, sorted again either alphabetically or according to frequency of occurrence, and made available as a file or a printout.

Difference Between Vocabularies A and B (A3)

Vocabulary X is determined. It consists of all pairs of elements contained in vocabulary A but not in vocabulary B.
For example, given the vocabularies A = (I, 3; you, 7; he, 5; she, 8) and B = (she, 2; we, 1) vocabulary C then contains C = (I, 3; you, 7; he, 5)

Furthermore, it is also possible to determine the limited difference between the vocabularies. In other words, vocabulary X may include pairs of elements which have the same word forms and which appear in both vocabularies if the ratio between the frequency of a word's occurrence in vocabulary B to that in vocabulary A does not exeed a specified value. Thus in the example, the pair (she, 8) belongs to vocabulary X given a limiting value of R = 0.25.

Intersection of Vocabularies A and B (A4)

Vocabulary X is determined. It consists of all pairs of elements present in both vocabularies A and B (possibly with different frequencies of occurrence). The frequency for a pair in vocabulary X is the sum of the frequencies in A and B.

Application of Dictionary D to Vocabulary A (A5)

Applying dictionary D to vocabulary A produces a distribution of the categories in vocabulary A and an internal differentiation of each category.
For example, with dictionary D = (cut_off, Castration; knife, Castration; judgement, Guilt) and vocabulary A = (cut_off, 4; knife, 4; judgement, 2) we have the relation X = (cut_off, Castration, 4; knife, Castration, 4; judgement, Guilt, 2). This produces the selections S_1 = (Castration, 8) and S_2 = (Guilt, 2). This example is presented in Table 3.1.

Word Form	Category	h_{abs}	h_{rel}
cut_off	CASTRATION	4	0.4
knife	CASTRATION	4	0.4
		8	0.8
judgement	GUILT	2	0.2
		2	0.2
		10	1.0

Table 3.1 Example of the application of a dictionary to a vocabulary

Comment: The concepts "relation" and "selection" were taken from relation algebra following CODD (1979). This makes it possible to present the processing forms described here in a formal mathematical manner (not shown here for the sake of clarity).

3.3.2 Structure-Oriented Processing

Application of a Dictionary to a Text (A7)

Every word form in a text is searched in a dictionary and replaced by the appropriate category. Word forms not contained in the dictionary are replaced by the category "undefined". The product of this form of processing is a sequence of categories corresponding to the sequential structure of the text.

Processing a Sequence of Categories (A8)

With the aid of conditions and instructions it is possible to manipulate a sequence of categories. The following conditions are possible:

- The occurrence of a category within the sequence studied
- The position of a category within the sequence studied
- The relation to the categories preceding and following a category within the sequence studied
- The conjunction of two categories within the sequence studied

Where such conditions apply, one of the following instructions can be carried out:

D_1	WORD FORM	CATEGORY	D_2	WORD FORM	CATEGORY
	accusation	ATTACK LEGAL SIGN-REJECT		accusation	GUILT
	doctor	AUTH-THEME HIGHER STATUS MEDICAL		doctor	CASTRATION
	mother	FAMILY FEMALE-ROLE HIGHER STATUS		mother	SEPARATION
	broke	AVOID ECONOMIC		broke	SHAME
	rival	ASCEND-THEME ATTEMPT SIGN-REJECT		rival	CASTRATION
	worry	DISTRESS SIGN-WEAK		worry	GUILT
	appartment	FEMALE THEME SOCIAL PLACE		appartment	SEPARATION
	naked	DANGER-THEME SENSORY-REFERENCE SEX-THEME		naked	SHAME

X	CATEGORY IN D_2	CATEGORY IN D_1
	SHAME	AVOID ECONOMIC DANGER-THEME SENSORY-REFERENCE SEX-THEME
	CASTRATION	ASCEND-THEME ATTEMPT AUTH-THEME HIGHER STATUS JOB-ROLE MEDICAL SIGN-REJECT
	GUILT	ATTACK DISTRESS LEGAL SIGN-REJECT SIGN-WEAK
	SEPARATION	FAMILY FEMALE-ROLE FEMALE-THEME HIGHER STATUS SOCIAL PLACE

<u>Table 3.2</u> Example of evaluation of two dictionaries

- Addition of a category
- Deletion of a category
- Substitution of a category
- Printing of the text preceding and following a category

Interaction Sequences (A9)
Starting from a sequence of categories, it is possible to formalize the sequences of categories for a change in speakers and to analyze them with specially prepared models.

3.3.3 Summary of the Forms of Processing

It is possible to divide the methods for analyzing texts into two groups by distinguishing between quantity- and structure-oriented forms. Another criterium for classifying the methods is given by the possibility to analyze texts resulting from a conversational situation according to a monadic or dyadic approach.

In the monadic form, only the contribution of an individual speaker is used in the analysis. In the dyadic form, in contrast, especially those speech phenomena are taken into consideration that result from the interaction of all participating speakers. Thus four basic groups of methods can be distinguished in computer-aided text analysis:

	MONADIC	DYADIC
QUANTITY ORIENTED	Group 1	Group 2
STRUCTURE ORIENTED	Group 3	Group 4

The choice of one of these groups of methods depends on the goal of the research. In the following, several examples of applications are listed together with the group of methods which is especially appropriate.

Group 1
Alterations in a patient's speech in the course of psychotherapeutic treatment
Comparison of different forms of therapy

Comparison of different groups of patients

Group 2
Interaction sequences in the therapeutic dyad
Speaker typologies

Group 3
Structures of a patient's associations

Group 4
An analyst's interpretative strategies

Generally, methods from different groups are combined for more extensive kinds of questions in order to get results which are more reliable.

3.4 Special Features of Spoken Speech

Spoken speech diverges from written language in numerous ways. The following sections deal with two kinds of problems resulting from this divergence which are of special significance to computer-aided text analysis.

3.4.1 The Problem of Transcription

A large number of transcription systems have been published in the past 12 years. The most widespread are probably HIAT1 and HIAT2, by EHLICH and REHBEIN (1976, 1979), which today function as a kind of standard. The special interests concerning computer-aided analysis of transcribed texts are usually not taken into consideration. For example, it is exceptionally involved, if at all possible, to convert "score notation" for sequential processing by a computer. One of the few systems suitable for machine processing was developed by BAUSCH (1971); it was employed as early as 1971 for spoken standard language at the Institute of the German Language (IDS). Its use is restricted by the disadvantage that it starts from a concept of sentence that at the most can be found in a subset of the different types of texts in spoken speech, such as in lectures. In the therapeutic interview, where a great variability in language structure must be presumed, it is usually not possible to determine exact sentences. On the contrary, in this situation there are breaks in the flow of speech, and the text can be structured as cadences (see HENNE and REHBOCK 1979). Then, however, the period is no longer a punctuation mark in the traditional sense, but a notation marking the end of a cadence at the basic tone. This can have far-reaching consequences for a sentence-based form of linguistic data processing.

Further problems are associated with literary transcription. How can the LDP algorithms familiar to us deal with word forms such as "haves", "somethen", or "ya"? How should dialects or phenomena such as changes in speech be treated? The notation of the speech expression is of special significance (see WINKLER 1979, 1983). It has been recognized, for example, that it is not possible to evaluate whether the self-sentiment a speaker expresses in a text is positive or negative except by referring to notation for the stress or elongation given to a word form and to the distinction as to whether a cadence ends with a raised voice, level voice, or basic voice.

The transcription rules developed within the framework of the ULM TEXTBANK are able to solve some of these problems. They are based on the following seven principles, already discussed in Sect. 1.6:

1. Morphologic naturalness of the transcripts
2. Structural naturalness of the transcripts
3. Transcript as an exact reproduction
4. Universality of the transcription rules
5. Completeness of the system
6. Independence of the transcription rules
7. Intellectual elegance of the rules

While these are, of course, ideals which can never be completely attained, initial experience has shown that it is possible to employ the transcription system based on these ideals in work which is either clinical, such as in supervision, or scientific, whether with or without the aid of computers.

3.4.2 The Problem Posed by Lemmatization

The description of one of the better known procedures for automatic lemmatization - SALEM devised by EGGER's et al. (1980, p. 26) - contains a list of structural restrictions "that can lead to premature termination of the analysis and thus probably to insufficient lemmatization". These items are:

- Participial clauses
- Insertions in parentheses that are not complete sentences
- Incorrect punctuation
- Years (given in numbers)
- Words in appositions
- Direct speech
- Bracketing out of lists or words in appositions
- Incomplete sentences

This list could also be used without any problems to characterize typical features of spoken speech. This means that the lemmatization of verbatim protocols cannot be expected to be reliable. Another well-known procedure, the LEMMA system described by WILLEE (1979, 1982), is more encouraging. Its two components probably make it possible for the results for at least the part dealing with word forms (with exceptions concerning incomplete words, idiosyncrasies, and literary forms) to be comparable to those for written or standard language. However, the qualification mentioned above concerning the application of LEMMA to sentences probably also applies to SALEM.

It is obvious that further research is necessary in this connection. One suggestion would be to develop a more universal variant for the processing of sentences which could be described as context-related. BOOT (1976, 1977, 1978) introduced the concept of "pattern matching grammar" in this regard; its implementation in practice might lead one step further. Consideration should especially be given to the manner in which the additional information on speech expression that is provided by spoken speech in contrast to written language can be used adavantageously in lemmatization and especially in overcoming ambiguities. On the acoustical channel this information includes:

- Voice pitch
- Loudness
- Fullness of voice
- Timber
- Speed
- Rhythm
- Accents
- Articulation
- Style of speech
- Connotative form

and on the visual channel

- Interpretative aids
- Control features

(listed according to FÄHRMANN 1967, pp. 115-119). This indicates a new area of activity for linguistic data processing, which could be outlined as follows:

1. Basic study of the contribution with regard to

   a) the notation for speech expression
   b) paraverbal speech phenomena
   c) nonverbal speech phenomena

   in order to determine the word class and variants of meaning

2. Segmenting according to cadences as the natural limit on context-related analyses

3. Inclusion of speech phenomena such as

   incomplete words, repetitions, incomplete sentences, parapraxis, and incomprehensible speech

4. Setting an adequate standard for transcription

New areas of application are continuously arising for "context-related lemmatization of transcribed spoken speech". In the ULM TEXTBANK alone ten million words of running text have yet to be subject to a qualified computer-aided linguistic analysis.

3.5 Text Analysis and Minimal Text Size

If speech data are to be used in a scientific study to determine measurements, the question is quickly posed as to the selection of the appropriate sample. This question is important if for no other reason than because only a portion of a particular speaker's speech is available, which is especially true of analyses of conversations. There are two fundamental problems: the determination of the parent text population and that of a sample (see ALEKSEEV 1984 for the linguostatistic point of view). The former is necessary for reasons of economy in order to be able to utilize only a portion of the treatment sessions that actually take place in the study of clinical questions. For a discussion of this issue see KOPS (1977) or GRÜNZIG (1984). The latter aspect concerns the length of a section of text used in the analysis. This can be of significance, for example, in the decision as to whether single utterances or entire conversations should be used. There have not been any sound scientific studies on these questions. As far as the text size has been taken into consideration in published studies at all, the authors rely primarily on the observations that they were able to make while analyzing speech material. GOTTSCHALK and GLESER (1969) determine, for example, that their scales could be utilized to ascertain anxiety by means of content analysis for a (English) text of at least 70 words. SCHÖFER (1976a, b, 1977) gives 100 words as the minimum value for the German version of these scales. This minimum is founded methodologically in the reliability with which numerous evaluators were able to classify test sentences. RUOFF (1973) describes texts of 200 word forms as the minimum size which is also applicable in practice. He bases this on his view that phenomena necessary to speech are normally distributed; this normal distribution begins to occur in the corpus of spoken speech that he studied in southern Germany at this text length. These are wellfounded indications of minimum size for computer-aided text analysis; usually values between 500 and 1000 word forms are suggested without further discussion.

A way to estimate the necessary sample size will now be described for the methods mentioned above. It is a significant aid to practical work, especially to computer-aided content analysis.

The considerations given here start from the idea that the process of speech production in man can be understood as a stochastic process (see BENNET 1977). In other words, laws of probability describe the origin of a text and determine the sequence of the individual word forms in it. Although these laws are at first unknown, they can be discovered empirically. The following assumptions are therefore made:

1. In spoken communication between individuals, different speech situations can be defined, which are described by different laws of probability.

2. The sequence of all the word forms in a collection of texts from one speech situation, called text corpus for short, represents the laws of probability for that speech situation.

It is possible on this basis to determine the basic vocabulary of a text corpus. Statistically, the basic vocabulary can be understood as the parent population from which a concrete text is taken as a sample. The frequency of occurrence of individual word forms stored in the basic vocabulary can be viewed as their general probability of occurrence; it thus constitutes an empirically determined measurement of probability. The idea of a basic vocabulary is also used by HENKEN (1976) in a computer-aided content analysis of documents from people who attempted suicide. He comments with regard to sample size: "Each group contained a minimum of 1000 words to insure reliability" (p. 37). The values for different categories, determined using the Harvard Psycho-Sociological Dictionary, were compared with a baseline derived from a one-million-word corpus of American prose (KUCERA and FRANCIS 1967). The values for the proportions of the categories range in this study between 0.06% and 8.93%. To be able to compare the results for individual texts, the significant deviations from the baseline in both directions were determined for 0.1%, 1% and 5% probability of error. Not taken into consideration, however, was whether a significant deviation from the given probability of error is at all possible for a sample size of 1000 words and a, for example, 0.06% probability of error. In the following an estimate is derived for this case.

If we carry out the processing from A5 (for applying a dictionary to a vocabulary), as defined above, for any given dictionary on the basic vocabulary, we determine the probability of occurrence, population for each category, based on the empirically studied parent. If we now consider a text which we are to analyze to be an arbitrary sample from the above- mentioned population (which is obviously not the case because of syntactic conventions, but which can - at least from a quantity point of view - be assumed to be sufficient approximation), we can make statements about those deviations considered to be random from the parameter of the totality at a given probability of error a. The probability b that the event k_i occurs z times in n observations is

$$b = \binom{n}{z} p_i^z (1-p_i)^{n-z} \tag{3.1}$$

Since the number of events for each of the categories may be either more or less than the values expected on the basis of general probability, the lower limit z_u and the upper limit z_o can be calculated:

$$\sum_{z=0}^{z_u} b \leq \frac{a}{2} < \sum_{z=0}^{z_{u-1}} b \tag{3.2}$$

and

$$\sum_{z=z_o}^{n} b \leq \frac{a}{2} < \sum_{z=z_{o+1}}^{n} b \tag{3.3}$$

To make an estimate of the minimal sample size n_{min}, we start from the requirement that a more than random deviation from the general probability should be possible for each category studied. In other words, a non random interpretation should be possible for every possible number of events of a category, i.e., from z=o to z=n. One practical meaning of this requirement is, for example, that a construct to be analyzed can be defined by the occurrence of mutually exclusive categories. The probability that an event occurs exactly o times on n observations given a general probability p is

$$w^{(0)} = (1-p)^n. \tag{3.4}$$

At a given probability of error a and a two-tailed question, $w^{(o)}$ must thus be less than a/2 for each value of n. From the relationship

$$(1-p)^n < \frac{a}{2} \tag{3.5}$$

and because

$$\lim_{n \to \infty} (1-p)^n = 0 \qquad (3.6)$$

we have either

$$n > {}^{(1-p)}\log \frac{a}{2} \qquad (3.7a)$$

or

$$n > \frac{\ln \frac{n}{2}}{\ln (1-p)} \qquad (3.7b)$$

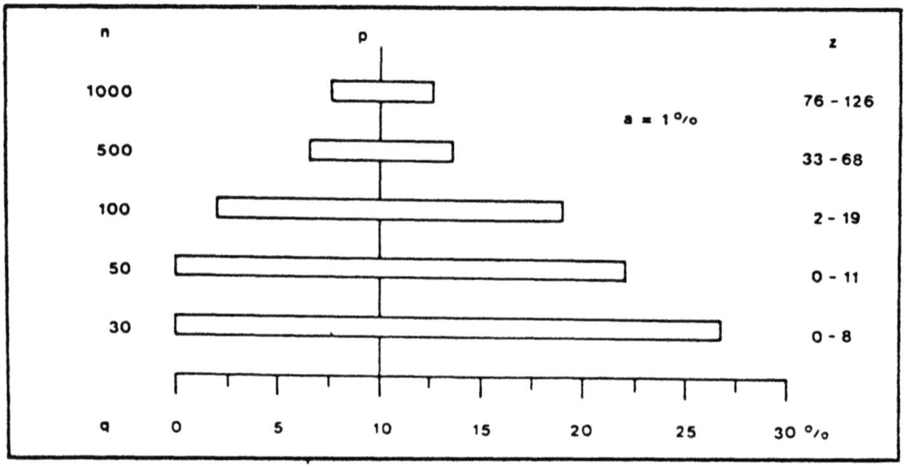

Figure 3.1 Confidence interval for the basic probability p=10% for different samples of size n and probability of error a=1%. The event numbers are given in absolute terms with z, in relative terms with q.

Figure 3.1 shows the dependence of z_u and z_o on sample size n for the probability p=10% and makes this result even clearer. If the value of n is less than the limiting value given by (3.7), the result can only be interpreted on one side, i.e., with regard to deviations above the limit. Yet even here there is only a limited range of variation, as shown in Fig. 3.1. The appendix to this study contains a table giving the minimal sample size for general probabilities between 0.01% and 10% for each of the common probabilities of error (1% and 5%). For the study by HENKEN mentioned above, this procedure demonstrates that the minimal sample size is 6146 words at a 5% probability of error for the category "medical", which has a general probability of 0.06%. Thus the 1000 words chosen by HENKEN are not sufficient to permit the findings to be interpreted.

Note: For some types of texts, such as conversations with a specialized vocabulary, it may be appropriate to employ the Poisson distribution instead of the binominal. In this case:

$$b = \frac{(pn)^k}{e^{pn}\ k!} \tag{3.8}$$

For the probability that the event occurs exactly o times,

$$w^{(0)} = \frac{1}{e^{pn}} \tag{3.9}$$

For the estimate of the lower limit,

$$\frac{a}{2} \geq e^{-pn} \tag{3.10}$$

or

$$n > - \frac{\ln \frac{a}{2}}{p} \tag{3.11}$$

3.6 Textbase Management System and Word Data Base

Numerous projects have been created within the scope of research of linguistic data processing and artificial intelligence in the past few years which are based in part on large text corpora. To a large extent, specialized computer-readable dictionaries have been developed, which emphasize different aspects of the stored word forms depending on the goal of the research. It is immediately obvious that the same intellectual effort has been made in different places; for example, a determination of the word kind for common word forms has certainly been performed hundreds of times. An obvious thought is to establish a central database for word forms where all important information can be collected and retrieved according to need. This idea has been raised by CALZOLARI (1983) for Italian and HEß et al. (1983) for German. The latter group, in a research project on the comparative analysis of computer-readable German texts, has concerned itself expecially with the problem of how the different forms of presentation employed in different computer-readable dictionaries can be transformed into a uniform structure. On the basis of this work, this group wants and has already begun to establish a "word data base for German" (BRUSTKERN et al. 1983, 1984; BRUSTKERN and SCHULZE 1983). The completion of this project would create an instrument for studying the German language which could without exaggeration be called unique. There are indications, however, as will be described below, that completion of this project will require a very long time.

The goal of the word data base for German is the cumulation of computer-readable German dictionaries. Initially a comparison of all the possible dictionaries was required, in order consequently to propose a "synthesis" for the structure of the word data base. This structure was arrived at in an impressive manner through the definition of so-called bit series; they make it possible to code entries on morphosyntactics, syntactic semantics, and pragmatics. Cumulation in the sense of these authors also refers to the computer-based transferral of word forms from the individual dictionaries into the structure of the word data base; it also refers to the adequate conversion of the information contained in the individual dictionaries. This goal itself, if nothing else, raises doubts about the success of the word data base, however. Since the process of making the individual dictionaries conform to the structure of the word data base can only be partially automatized, intellectual steps will have to be inserted and many compromises will have to be made. Thus, capitalization, umlauts, and multiple-word forms either were not or will not be incorporated into the word data base, according to the principle of employing the smallest possible denominator. From an economic point of view the question must be raised if it finally would not have been more sensible to undertake the development of a fundamentally new plan for all the word forms which are available, according to the features which can be coded with the bit series. This text should not be more difficult than the revision of the existing codes if a well-prepared menu technique were employed. Since no compromises would have to be made in this case, a qualitatively better product could also be expected. On the other hand, the total effort would not be inconsiderable since 14 man-years would be required given 300 thousand word forms and an estimated average processing time of 5 minutes per word form.

The question of whom this effort would finally serve is legitimate. At any rate, lexicographers would certainly not be among the potential users. They already posses a largest part of the information to be stored in the word data base for German. Yet, it would be interesting for projects such as the ULM TEXTBANK as an aid in the collection and editing of stored speech data. Thus the question as to whether the services of the word data base for German can already be utilized should be answered. During a visit to the IDS in the spring of 1984 it quickly became apparent that information other than just word kind is only available there for a small percentage of the 300 000 entries. If the fact is also taken into consideration that the possible advantages even for determination of word kind are also limited because of the compromises regarding capitalization and umlauts (both of which are standard elements at the ULM TEXTBANK to ensure user acceptance), there is no convincing reason for the services offered by the word data base to be used. The ULM TEXTBANK is not considering using them in its current work; on the contrary, it is continuing to establish the local word data base in Ulm. Care was taken in preparing its structure, however, so that the information it contains could be transferred to the word data base for German at a later date without any significant alterations.

3.6.1 The Ulm Word Data Base

The Ulm word data base is based on the idea of the basic vocabulary, which for the past 5 years has recorded all the word forms registered in the ULM TEXTBANK together with their frequencies of occurrence. For the past 2 years, the type and lemma have been determined for all the new word forms encountered during routine text corrections. This work is done at a visual display unit, and only the word forms to be treated by a processor appear on the screen. As an additional aid, the processor also has a printout of the text in which the word forms to be processed are printed in red. This ensures that the word types can be determined functional-syntactically, and the lemmata in a context-related manner. It is intended that the homographs be resolved during the text correction procedure which will accompany the planned migration of the ULM TEXTBANK from a TR440 to the successor Siemens, model 7550 D.

Further information on word types is coded columnwise on paper and input in a rational way for a larger amount of new word forms at irregular intervals. In this manner, it is possible to code an average of two words per minute. The features to be coded were selected taking into account the hypotheses mentioned in sect. 1.2.3 and their verifiability.

3.6.2 Structure and Design of the Word Data Base

The Ulm word data base is divided logically into two collections:

- Index of lemma names
- Index of complete forms

Lemma names and complete forms are linked together so that the lemma name can be found for each complete form and, vice versa, all complete forms can be found for each lemma name.

The most important rule for lemmatization is the observance of consistency with regard to word kind (parts of speech) and word meaning. The elements in the catalogues of features for the ULM TEXTBANK are as follows:

LEMMA NAME

1 graphemic presentation of the lemma name
2 identification of a lemma's variant meanings
3 reference to corresponding complete forms
4 semantic description (planned)
5 frequency of occurrence of all examples of a lemma
6 information on the lemma's grammar

WORD KIND

1	noun	7	negation
2	verb	8	article
3	adjective	9	preposition
4	adverb	10	conjunction
5	pronoun	11	interjection
6	numeral	12	other

MORPHOLOGY OF LEMMA

1 simplex
2 compound
3 derivative of prefix or suffix
4 derivative of stem
5 derivative of adjective
6 derivative of infinitive
7 numbers used nominally
8 abbreviation
9 personal name
10 multiple-word form

	WORD ORIGIN		GENDER (in German)		PARTICIPLE VERB (in German)
1	foreign word	1	masculin	1	have
2	dialect	2	feminine	2	be
		3	neutral		

COMPLETE FORMS

1 graphemic presentation of the complete form
2 identification of the variant meanings of the complete form
3 reference to corresponding lemma names
4 semantic description (planned)
5 frequency of occurrence of all examples of a complete form
6 information on the grammar of the complete form
see the folowing lists.

	RELATIVE FORMS		NUMBERS
1	diminutive	1	singular
2	comparative	2	plural
3	superlative	3	plural only

	MORPHOLOY FOR COMPLETE FORM		CASE/MODE
1	present participle	1	nominative/indicative
2	past participle	2	genitive/conjunctive
3	present tense	3	dative/imperative
4	past tense	4	accusative
5	infinitive with "to"		

3.6.3 Size of the Word Data Base

The Ulm word data base currently comprises approximately 85_000 German entries. Almost half of these are lemmata. Tables 3.3 and 3.4 provide details on some of the features listed above for the 57_000 word forms already processed. An English version of the Ulm word data base has recently been started and actually comprises 25_000 entries.

PART OF SPEECH	abs	rel	PART OF SPEECH	abs	rel
noun	26463	46.4	negation	4	0.0
verb	17217	30.2	article	16	0.0
adjective	11147	19.5	preposition	73	0.1
adverb	788	1.4	conjunction	151	0.3
pronoun	239	0.4	interjection	88	0.2
numerals	476	0.8	other	426	0.8

Table 3.3 Distribution of the parts of speech in the Ulm word data base

	noun	verb	adj.	adv.
MORPHOLOGY				
simplex	14.6	24.7	41.2	22.6
compound word	51.9	4.5	9.3	62.6
pre/suffix	11.2	62.2	17.0	2.8
root	6.5		32.0	11.5
ETYMOLOGY				
foreign	30.5	8.2	23.7	8.8
dialect	1.1	7.3		
GRADATION/DIMINUITION				
diminutive	1.0			
comparative	0.3		1.8	0.8
superlative	0.4		1.7	3.4

Table 3.4 Distribution of selected features for four word kinds from the Ulm word data base; in percent/word kind and group

4 The Text Base Management System: Information Science Applied in the Field of Psychotherapy

The previous chapters have dealt with psychotherapeutic research employing language data and thus with the general scope of application of linguistic data processing and with the questions associated with it. This chapter will discuss the details of several aspects that were important for the actual establishment of the TBS. This chapter contributes to applied information science, demonstrating which elements from the current state of research have been employed in practical work at the TBS. However, there have also been some rather severe limitations, since hardly any software tools were available with the computer at the University Computer Center in Ulm (a TR440 will be in use until probably mid-1985). Because, on the other hand, the planned change in computers was originally scheduled for 1982, the few tools which were available were not given serious consideration with regard to the establishment of the TBS because they are highly machine dependent. Due to the lack of hard- and software capacity, a number of problems were solved "only" on paper or were solved in a preliminary way, in the sense of "rapid prototyping" (KEUTGEN 1982), by using the microcomputer equipment (Telecomp 5200 and 5600) at our disposal, in order to make the system available to users.

4.1 Scientific Features of the TBS

The concept of text base system, which has been used descriptively until now, is defined and given substance in this section. The first step is the introduction of definitions to distinguish the members in this family of information systems. Following that, the TBS in Ulm is contrasted with the development of other existing or planned comparable systems.

4.1.1 Definitions

The documents stored in the ULM TEXTBANK are a collection consisting primarily of open text corpora. The characteristic of an **open corpus** is that it is an excerpt from a parent population which is continuously being expanded without being tied to the goal of completeness. An example is the collection of completely transcribed short psychotherapies. It is possible to expand this corpus to include every newly undertaken treatment without ever reaching a state of completeness or representativeness with regard to the text type "short psychotherapy". The quality of **completeness** can only be approximated if there are features limiting the composition of the corpus. Thus a collection of diagnostic first interviews has a higher degree of completeness if it consists of equal parts on the features "sex", "age", "diagnosis", and "social strata". An example of a completely closed corpus is the Bible (see PARUNAK 1982).

The degree of completeness exhibited by a corpus also influences the strategies for handling the results of text analyses. There are two principal approaches. In the one, all the available results of analyses are stored completely with the text or in direct relation to the text. In the other, parts of the corpus are processed algorithmically as needed. As detailed by PARUNAK (1982, p. 150), users with open corpora tend to use the algorithmic version, while the storage of existing results from previous studies is often preferred for closed corpora. According to the theory of science this is because research on closed corpora is usually comparative. Open corpora constitute a sample and are employed to test or generate hypotheses. In addition, they are usually only analyzed once, in contrast to closed corpora which often have a very long history as objects of scientific interest, as clearly shown by research on the Bible or Goethe's work. This also explains why closed corpora were stored electronically much earlier than open corpora, while the latter are still sometimes treated as a disposable product. The example of research on psychotherapeutic talks indicates how the introduction of the concept of text bank and the accompanying technology first made it possible to recognize the spread of multiple use of one and the same data set to answer different scientific questions.

The consequence for the ULM TEXTBANK - as a collection of primarily open corpora - is that it makes text analysis available by means of algorithmic editing. Yet with regard to one of its goals, namely to open possibilities for the multiple analysis of language data gained with great effort, the plan is for the TBS to be able to store results directly with the texts. The following tasks are consequently posed to a system intended to manage a text bank:

1. Input and editing of texts according to numerous points of view.

2. Management of an unlimited number of text units on the computer center's auxiliary storage.

3. Management of an unlimited amount of information on the text units, their authors, and the related text analyses.

4. Management of an open quantity of methods for editing and analyzing stored text units.

5. Assistance for interfaces to statistical and other user packages.

6. Assistance for a simple, dialogue-oriented user interface when the texts mentioned in points 1 to 5 are supplied or performed.

The tasks mentioned in point 1 belong to the domain of text processing. The term **text processing system** can be used if sufficient user assistance is provided.

The task of managing an unlimited number of text units on an auxiliary storage (point 2) is the object of long-term data maintenance. The stored sets are grouped in files and put in magnetic storage. If, in addition, it is possible to administer the data sets with the access methods provided by the operating system, then it is possible to speak of a data maintenance system or a **file management system** (e.g., Archive with BS2000 from Siemens and Datatrieve with VMS from Digital Equipment).

The tasks mentioned in point 3 concern the management of a data base including all of its services. These tasks are fulfilled by general **data base management systems**; the classic functions of such system are the description, handling, take up, manipulation, and retrieval of data. Data structures can be classified as hierarchic, network oriented, or relational.

Point 4 refers to a collection of methods that, given computer assistance in the user's selection of methods, can be termed a method base. Further assistance, such as method documentation and parameter input, it is provided by the **method base management system.** Point 5, on interfaces, is a subset of the tasks described by point 4.

All of these tasks are collected in point 6 with regard to the user interface. Thus the TBS is an integrated overall system consisting of

file management system	(FMS)
data base management system	(DBMS)
text management system	(TMS)
method base management system	(MBMS)

Since the selection of the specific data to be managed by the DBMS and of the methods provided by the MBMS is made in accordance with the kind of texts managed by the FMS, it is legitimate to describe the overall information system as tailor-made. The following definition of the entire system is made, in analogy to the definitions of the individual components, in order to ensure that our terminology adequately reflects this state of affairs:

Text bank management system - TBMS
Branch: Linguistic data processing

The TBMS is an information system that can administer texts and information on texts, and that makes texts accessible by integrating techniques from linguistic data processing and text processing. It features a homogeneous user interface that assists in the take up, processing, output, and analysis of text units.

As mentioned previously, the shorter phrase "Text bank system" (TBS) is used at the ULM TEXTBANK.

The TBMS differs from document retrieval systems by containing two additional components: text processing and method base. It is true that the emphasis, as far as retrieval in the TBMS is concerned, is still on data retrieval (for requests made according to the author of a text) and on document retrieval (for text references to be determined according to text-immanent features). Fact retrieval is nonetheless an integral component of all the plans for a TBMS, even if systems able to cope with large quantities of material from colloquial speech are still not ready for production. Ideally this should not be a basis for differentiating within a TBMS anyway. "The demand that both kinds of retrieval be integrated in one system is repeated again and again because it comes closer to actual practice" (JOCHUM 1980, p. 124). This is a sentence that deserves to be emphasized.

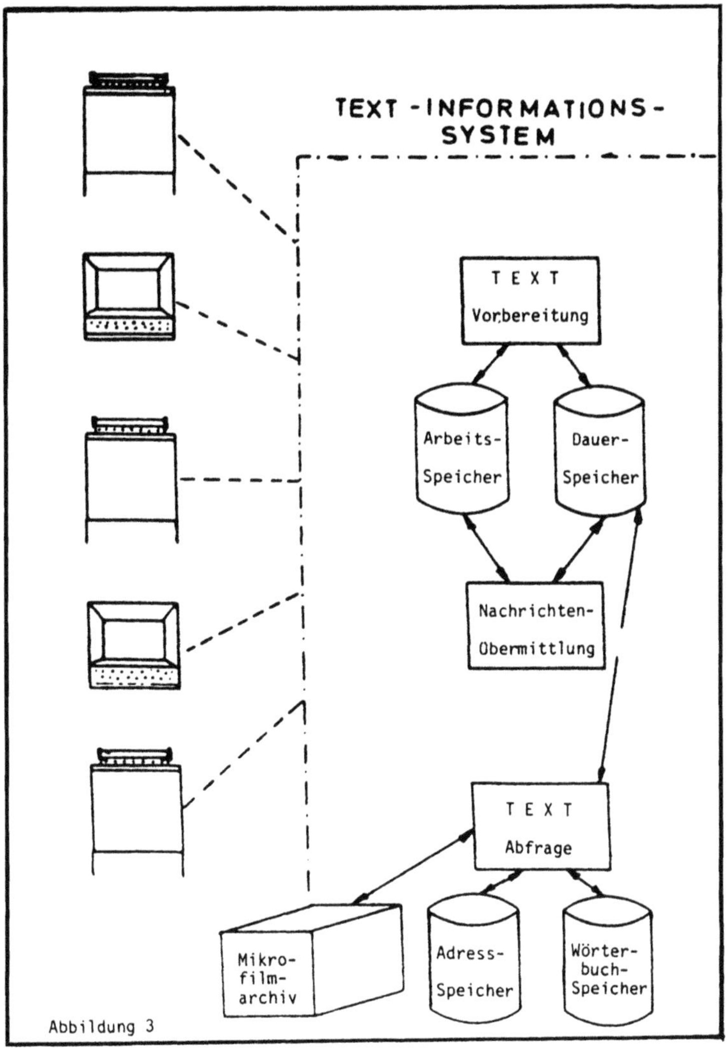

Figure 4.1 "Text Bank System" after DÜRR (1970, p.313)

4.1.2 Comparable Systems and Approaches

In data processing, the maintenance of complete documents as data does not have a long tradition, although it is true that texts have been edited and processed almost as long as electronic data processing has existed. An early example is the text information system (presented by DÜRR 1970) for managing texts in a microfilm archive (Fig. 4.1). The idea of a text base analogous to a data base and with corresponding support facilities was first raised for German at the end of the 1970s. Independently of one another, systems satisfying the definition of TBMS given above were conceived at the Max Planck Institute for History in Göttingen, the Department of Psychotherapy at the University of Ulm (both at the end of 1978), and the Sociology Department at the University of Bielefeld (at the end of 1979). These projects have been reported to a wider scientific audience in a number of publications (MERGENTHALER 1979, 1981, 1983, 1984; MERGENTHALER and KÄCHELE 1983; THALLER 1980a, 1982, 1983a,b,c, 1984; PAULUS 1984). No development of such systems has been reported from the Anglo-Saxon world, the reason probably being the different manner of funding research in the social sciences, where the need for a TBMS has been the greatest. For example, the problem of obtaining extensive access to computers is an insurmountable financial barrier for American colleagues doing psychotherapy research. One consequence is that text data from Philadelphia and San Francisco are being temporarily stored in Ulm within the framework of cooperative research projects. The same is true in Göttingen with regard to historical data.

Aspects of Individual Systems or Solutions

Development of the system **CLIO** was initiated at the Max Planck Institute for History in Göttingen at the end of 1978. The aim was to prepare a general, data base oriented program system "which should be in a position to assist in as many forms of editing and for as many different types of historical sources as possible" (THALLER 1984, p. 98). In addition, the practical demand was raised that the original nature of a source should be retained, independent of the analyses to be conducted, so that the user interface is comparable with that of the common statistical packages, such as the SPSS, and presupposes as little knowledge of the local operating system as possible. The current status of this project is a complex system containing all the components of a TBMS (see the CLIO user handbook, THALLER 1982, 1983a, and the CLIO introduction and summary, THALLER 1983b).

The user of CLIO is largely freed of the task of the administration of text sources. This is accomplished by putting the entire document including an unlimited number of descriptive features on a system file and transferring it to the auxiliary storage. The special strength of CLIO is, however, the data base, which permits comprehensive research in the Text Bank starting from descriptive features. The possibilities to choose from are oriented toward the types of questions customary in historical research and toward the pecularities of the material. An example is the presentation of dates in the German, American, Latin, and revolutionary forms, that CLIO can interpret in their temporal relationship. Another prominent feature is the capacity to process incomplete information and inexact values (THALLER 1984).

Less developed in the current version of CLIO is the method base. The possibilities in this regard are limited to the simpler procedures of linguistic data processing, content analysis, and editing. However, further development according to which extensive string manipulations are supposed to be introduced already being prepared. This change will make it possible not only to lemmatize, but also to use an improved search language in order "to use the language content of an unlimited context, expressed in a word-oriented file, to jump back into the data base system that the relevant texts are from, and to conduct further specific data base activities there" (THALLER 1983, p. 265).

CLIO's user interface is language oriented (i.e., based on elements from the Romance languages). No use is made of the opportunities provided by menu and mask techniques to guide the user. The system is implemented with FORTRAN, ASSEMBLER, and PL/1 on a Univac 1100. The planned development of CLIO also means making the system more portable.

In contrast to CLIO, whose general aims make it an instrument for many divers projects, the program system **Textan** (PAULUS 1984) was developed especially for a research project in the social sciences. Numerous interviews constitute the data to be managed and evaluated with the aid of a computer. Its plan also called for an integrated interaction of the modules typical for a TBMS. These modules were implemented employing predominantly producer-specific software (TR440).

The data acquisition in this project took place on the OCR/A document reader soft- and hardware at the ULM TEXTBANK. With regard to the method base, Textan is also limited to the simpler methods of linguistic data processing. Although the project has been completed in the meantime, the Textan program system will not be used any more because it is highly machine dependent.

In addition to these two systems and that of the ULM TEXTBANK described in this study, which all follow the integrated approach of file, data base, and method base management systems, there have also been a number of other attempts which, in very different ways, have emphasized and realized individual aspects of a TBMS. In the following, a few typical examples are briefly discussed.

SCHUPP (1984, p. 96) reports the development of a text management system (**TMS**) "as an aid in the economic management of texts on the basis of interactions.... It should make it possible for an organizational system designed to classify a text on a substantive basis to be handled in a flexible manner. Furthermore, it should guarantee the capacity to retrieve information (also in context) at any time". The main emphasis of the TMS is on a greatly improved editing component; with it a text can also be coded before it is stored in the text bank. The texts can be recorded and printed according to these codes. A distinct data base component providing the possibility of retrieving individual objects is not included.

DEGENHARDT and DEGENHARDT (1984) have undertaken the attempt to reach a solution similar to TBMS by means of a commercially available data base system (**SIR**, STATUS Corp., Berlin). They divided the text into lines, numbered them, and stored them along with further information in the data base system as simple data. By using the line number as a search label it is possible to retrieve texts according to other features with the aid of a search language. This approach has been proven to be impractical for larger amounts of text.

The approach followed by STONEBRAKER et al. (1983) is also based on a data base system. Starting with **INGRES** (HELD et al. 1975; STONEBRAKER et al. 1976), they developed a proposal for managing documents within the framework of a relational data base. Their proposal amounts to introducing data elements in the form of strings of variable length and making the corresponding string operations available. The advantage of this solution is that text access is very simple and user oriented.

This approach is well suited for closed corpora, even those larger in size. PARUNAK (1982) has demonstrated this for the Bible, as mentioned above.

GASS et al. (1983) have used a documentation system (**STAIRS**, IBM 1972) to manage a dream data base (DDB). Individual dreams, together with descriptive features, are input into the data base in the same way as documents. Selection according to specific criteria is possible via the retrieval language. Substantive dream analysis is achieved by inserting intellectually prepared codes into the dream text; these codes can later be used as selection criteria.

The **MINDOK** system (INFODAS 1983) puts the emphasis on the document input phase. Along with extensive plausibility tests for the data describing the documents, the spelling of the clear text is checked using user-specific dictionaries. Moreover, data and documents are stored in a common data base, as in the previous example. MINDOK does not have a method base; an interface, however, is to be installed to enable users to employ their own text analysis programs.

The **MIDOC** system follows similar goals (KOWARSKI and MICHAUX 1983). It has distinct text processing and data base components. It was conceived for office use and implemented on a microcomputer. Text analysis methods are therefore not provided.

The aims of the **SONIS** system are entirely different (STELCK 1984). Its three main components are the data base, method base, and model base systems. The data base component is based on the relational model. The texts are not implemented as data types and, consequently, can only be edited in the same manner as that used by PARUNAK (see above). In contrast, the method base component of SONIS is all the more flexible. It now includes the model component, which here refers to the problem-specific determination of applicable methods, the execution of the methods, and the permissibility of the data.

Another approach is that customary in the systems designed for computer-aided content analysis. In **LDVLIB** (DREWEK and ERNI 1982) and **TEXTPACK** (MOHLER and ZUELL 1984), texts are stored in system files together with identifying features. By referring to the identifiers it is possible to compile subcorpora from the system files. TEXTPACK also offers the capacity to link any data file and the system text file in order to select texts according to other criteria. On the other hand, this type of system has a distinct method base component; this is especially true of the LDVLIB. The data base and, in TEXTPACK, the file management play, in contrast, a subordinate role, if any at all.

The Archive Retrieval and Analysis System **ARRAS** (SMITH 1984) is a well suited text analysis system for large texts. It works on a text base but does not support a data base component.

4.1.3 Possible Application of TBMS

In principle, a TBMS can be employed anywhere a large number of texts are created or required and are not only to be used once. This opens a wide spectrum of applications, e.g., in offices and publishing houses, in government agencies and hospitals, and in universities. In fact, however, the text bank idea is just gradually appearing in all of these areas. To give one example, KNAUEL (1982) puts a question mark after the heading "Magical Term 'Text Bank'" of his article on book production in the 1980s; similarly, at the Ninth International Conference on Very Large Data Bases, held in Florence in 1983, a panel met to discuss "Complex Data Objects: Text, Voices, Images: Can DBMS Manage Them?" This year a conference is being held for the first time which is concerned exclusively with the problem of **source base**; in this case source base refers to a generalization of the TBMS type system, including not only texts but other complex **data objects** as well, such as language and pictures. Source base will be a highlight at the Fifth International Conference on Data Base in the Human and Social Sciences, to take place in the United States in 1985. These examples demonstrate that information science is just beginning to concern itself with an area that has existed for users for several years.

A completely new field in this regard is the office and administration sector (CROFT and PEZARRO 1982). In the next few years there will be a flood of documents, created by the economically priced text processing systems, for which management aids are usually not present. A TBMS would certainly be a valuable instrument for gaining control over the mountains of diskettes surrounding many automatic text processors and filling many cabinets.

4.2 Software Technology and TBS

This section deals first with general points of view regarding the software development methodology, then with the methods used to design the TBS, and finally briefly with several aspects of software ergonomy.

4.2.1 Design Methodology

The history of the software design methods goes back to the late 1960s. BÖHM and JACOPINI demonstrated at that time that it is possible to write programs based solely on logical control structures. Specifically, they distinguished between sequence, binary decisions, and loop formation. Not much later DIJKSTRA (1968a, 1968b, 1970, 1972) developed his ideas concerning the "GOTO", disclosing it to be a source of error and proposing structured programming as an alternative. WIRTH (1971) worked in the same direction. Mills worked out the mathematical bases of these developments by combining the ideas of DIJKSTRA, BÖHM, and JACOPINI. He thus initiated a change during which the methodology of programming increasingly developed from an individual art to an engineering activity (see TAUSWORTHE 1977, p. 99ff.; see EGGELING 1984 for a critical examination from the perspective of industrialization). NASSI and SHNEIDERMAN (1973) recommended **structograms** as a means of presentation; which now have achieved wide use in practical work with structured programs. Practical aids and ideas which have developed out of structograms are decision tables, normed programming, the pseudocode, and programming aids for applying structured programs.

In the following years software development became increasingly aware of another problem, which TAUSWORTHE termed the "development gap" (see Fig. 4.2). This gap is between the suggested problem-oriented solution and the possible machine-oriented solution. "Structured design methods are the attempt to bridge this gap. In this sense they are potentially much more important for the data processing user than just programming in sequential, selective, and rerun structures" (SNEED 1979, p. 718). A wealth of **software design methods** were created in 1975-1979 by adding instructions, procedure plans, and symbols to the structograms. Some of the best known are hierarchical input-processing output (HIPO, IBM 1975), structured analysis and design technique (SADT, Infotech 1978; COMBELIC 1978), JACKSON's system development (JSD, JACKSON 1983), information systems work and analysis of changes (ISAC, LUNDEBERG et al. 1979) and NIJSSEN's information analysis methodology (NIAM, VERHEIJEN and VAN BEKKUM 1982). For further information see BLANCK and KRIJGER (1983) or SCHULTZ (1982).

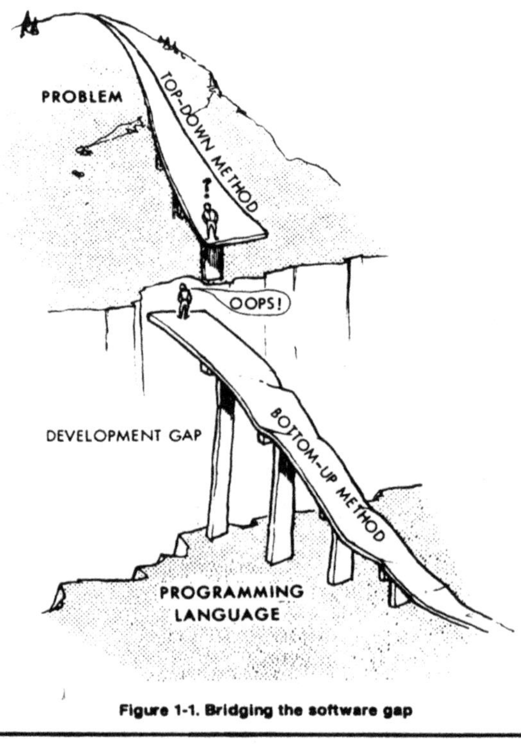

Figure 1-1. Bridging the software gap

Figure 4.2 "Development Gap" after TAUSWORTHE (1977, p.6)

A first attempt was undertaken to make a comparative evaluation of software design methods at a conference in the Netherlands in 1982 and a year later in England (OLLE et al. 1982, 1983). In order to make a comparison, the organizers of the first conference gave a standard application for which the authors of the individual methods were supposed to present suggested solutions. This attempt was only a partial success because it soon became apparent that not all the possibilities offered by the individual methods could be convered by the application of standard cases. At the second conference the analysis of individual components was therefore emphasized more strongly; this, however, pushed the comparative perspective into the background. MADDISON et al. (1983) discussed such comparative efforts critically. They contrasted eight methods by making a statement about each of them for more than 40 features. Yet the significance of this study is less the collection of these features than the conclusions that the authors drew from their analysis of the material. Three of these conclusions will be mentioned here. MADDISON et al. established, for example, that almost all design methods are still in the state of development. The consequence is that **no standard** had been established, at least by 1983. They also ascertained that most methods strongly rely on an **intuitive access** to the analysis and design process. "The phases and tasks which form the methodology are described in terms of 'what' should be done and rarely, if ever, in terms of 'how' they should be done" (MADDISON 1983, p. 99). Their third conclusion was a suggestion that the authors of design methods name the range, aims, philosophy, presuppositions, and expectations that their methods are based on. On this basis it could make sense to gather user's actual experiences and to measure them against the aims of the methods and of the expectations of the users.

The present trend in design methods aims at embedding them in a **software development environment**. In this sense the proposed computer-aided programming-(problem-solving) support system from Actis (Compact, Actis Corp., Stuttgart) would support the following areas:

- System description, development, and consistency test
- Check on terminology
- Design of data base and file structures
- Generation of functioning programs to administer the master data
- Generation of a report writer
- Generation of dialogue programs
- Generation of file converter programs
- Generation of standard processing routines

- Documentation accompanying the entire problem-solving process

The *ISAC-(information flow symbols for applied computer technology) methods constitute an implementation of the first element on this list (JOCHUM and WINTER 1981; GERKENS and WINTER 1984). They are a modification of the plan proposed by LUNDEBERG et al. (1979; the Actis version is identified here with an asterisk); "the elements for the presentation were reduced to two kinds and the procedure was simplified methodologically" (Actis, p. 6). This made it possible at the same time, to provide a theoretical foundation for the procedure by using the instance/channel interpretation of the Petri nets (GODBERSEN 1983, pp. 4-63).

SCHULTZ (1982b) suggests the term "computer-aided software design" (CAS) as a methodological procedure for software production environments. GOTTHARD et al. (1984) have also used this term for their "integrated methods for software design ANIMOS". They place three requirements on modern software engineering:

1. Symmetric view of functions and data
2. Covering the developmental phases
3. Imbedding in a software development environment

Consistently left out of consideration in all of these software design methods has been the future user of the software to be developed. Therefore a fourth requirement will be added here:

4. Orientation toward a user model

In the past few years the experience has often been made that the introduction of information systems in large plants and agencies is accompanied by general problems and especially by problems in staff behavior. It is not unusual for such problems to lead to a complete financial disaster. DAGWELL and WEBER (1983) give as one of the reasons for this change in behavior that system designers have an incorrect model of users. It seems to them that designers view users of information systems as individuals who require order and guidance in their lives and who are more interested in financial rewards than in increasing their personal esteem. "Thus, the designers may design tightly structured systems that lower the quality of working life and produce, as a consequence, the behavioral problems observed" (DAGWELL and WEBER 1983, p. 987). Referring to HEDBERG and MUMFORD (1975) and LUCAS (1975), DAGWELL and WEBER distinguished between two user images:

Theory X: Individuals who love order and desire no personal resonsibility for their own actions

Theory Y: Individuals who are responsible and prefer a kind of work which is full of variety

It can be assumed that designers following a theory X user model prepare tightly structured system designs, while, in contrast, designers with a theory Y user model design systems which make work more fulfilling. Low-quality work can be associated with the former type of system, high-quality work with the latter. Empirical investigations have shown that these distinctions can be very meaningful. For example, transcultural differences have been demonstrated; system designers in Australia and Sweden are oriented more toward theory Y, while Americans and English tend more to theory X. These results still have to be regarded as preliminary, however, because a large number of subordinate questions are still unanswered, such as whether the user model of a designer is constant over time, or whether the group of users is homogeneous with regard to theory X or Y.

This raises the following questions with regard to software design methods: Do methods like HIPO, which distinguish only between function and data, lead to theory X designs, while methods like ISAC, which also distinguish between person and material flows, to theory Y? If this question is considered under the impression of the results presented by DAGWELL and WEBER, this might lead to an explanation for the fact that the ISAC method was developed in Sweden and the HIPO in the United States.

4.2.2 Design and Representation of Software Architectures

The design method DRS (design and representation of software architecture) is presented in this section in the form it was applied in the development of the TBS. It is a procedure that originated in practical work and is based in ISAC and earlier work in the research group on computer-aided information systems at the Technical University of Berlin. The reason for describing this procedure is not a desire to present still another method, but is the fact that the methods mentioned in the previous section (this does not apply for *ISAC) are in general too powerful for small and medium-sized projects and tend to overload the representation and design process in low-complexity systems with ballast. A minimal framework will be described here which closes the gap between a program's planned course and ingenious development methodology for software tools; it thus makes it possible to reach operable designs in daily work quickly. The aims set for DRS were:

- Freedom for creativity in designing
- Prototyping as an integral part of the design process
- Software tools as an integral part of the design
- Computer aid in the design process

System design is first and foremost a creative process. Design methods can aid this process by providing descriptive means which can be learned quickly and are easy to employ, and by representing work techniques which make it possible or easier to find ideas (KOBERG and BAGNALL 1976). The design process is obstructed if a development methodology prescribes descriptive means which are difficult to grasp cognitively and are highly specific. Similarly, procedural design techniques inhibit creativity. For these reasons, DRS provides for only a few descriptive elements and rules.

An example is the dictionary top down vs. bottom up, which was the subject of some controversy in the past years. DRS supports, as its goal, a design corresponding to the top down principle. Finding the design can be, however, an iterative process between top down and bottom up, i.e., middle out.

Another example is module size. No exact answer is given here, either; the size of a simple module should result from its context in the overall plan. The commonly mentioned reason for using small modules, that is large modules are more susceptible to making errors, is unfounded, as BASILI and PERRICONE (1984) have shown. On the contrary, "the larger the module, the less error prone it was" (BASILI and PERRICONE 1984, p. 49). It is clear from their studies that the frequency of error increases with the inexactness of an interface description or parameter definition. But the implication of this for interfaces in a system design is that the more naturally the interfaces result from the overall design, the more exactly they can be described. Mistakes can thus be avoided.

Prototyping as an integral part of the development cycle can produce a number of advantages (see DEARNLEY and MAYHEW 1983). However, prototyping is almost essential if the potential users of the system to be developed are not well known or even still have to be found or motivated. Another situation which can be a cogent reason for using "rapid" prototyping is one that research projects are often in: the parallel course of production and development. Both of these reasons were true for the development of the TBS, so that a virtue was made of necessity.

Software tools are especially necessary as an integral part of the design being worked on if the requirements to be placed on the production system are not known in all details. This was the case for the TBS in several places, such as at the interface to text input or with the methods for text analysis that had to be integrated. However, these tools should be distinguished from those that are not an integral part of the design itself, but are aids in the preparation of the design; examples are interactive graphic tools and programming aids (see, e.g., INCE 1983).

Description of the Procedure

The DRS procedure requires that a system analysis has been made, which can be available either in its entirety (as according to WEDEKIND 1973), or only in its results, such as a notebook of requirements (DANIELS 1984). A design based on this approach is composed of the following parts:

1. Representation
   a) general
   b) detailed

2. Description
   a) static
   b) dynamic
   c) precedences

Representation
The representation part comprises graphic elements; with their aid the design is developed step by step and finally represented. Function diagrams of the current status aid in the **general representation** (see HAAG 1981, pp. 124ff.). The overall system can and should be organized into several levels of abstraction (on the use of the term abstraction see INHETVEEN and LUFT 1983, p.p. 544-545). The elementary parts of the general representation form the starting point for the **detailed representation**. This is prepared preferably with the aid of structograms (according to NASSI and SHNEIDERMAN 1973); the additions suggested by BÖCKMANN (1983) can also be employed. A detailed representation is not necessary, however; this is especially the case if programming tools are available (RAMSEY et al. 1983; ROOME 1979).

Table 4.1 provides a survey of the five different types of descriptive elements in the DRS. Included for each element are a long and a short designation, a symbol, and several examples.

The Static Element. All kinds of states, such as objects, circumstances, and information, are described by the static element, which can be either a data source or a data sink. It is characterized by a caption written in the oval symbol. Furthermore, elementary and nonelementary static elements are distinguished. An elementary static element cannot or should not be further subdivided within a system architecture; instead, it is put into the descriptive part. Nonelementary static elements combine several static elements, thus contributing to the clarity of representation. Since we are dealing with abstractions, they are not put into the descriptive part, but are further subdivided within the representative part down to their most elementary constituents.

The Dynamic Element. The description of events takes place by means of a dynamic element. Its designation is given next to the symbol used in the graphic representation. An elementary dynamic element cannot or should not be further subdivided within a system architecture; instead, its performance, features, and requirements are recorded in the descriptive part. A nonelementary dynamic element is an abstraction of several dynamic elements and can contain, in contrast to static elements, all other descriptive elements. Nonelementary dynamic elements are not put into the descriptive part.

No.	Designation		Symbol	Examples
1	static element	SE	⬭	count questionnaire computer printout file data base
1.1	nonelementary			
1.2	elementary		as 1.1	
2	dynamic element	DE		machine a step in work process program system
2.1	nonelementary		□	
2.2	elementary		■	
3	persons	P	◇	special assistant doctor programmer user typist
4	relation	R		
4.1	reading/writing	RW	———	print
4.2	communicating	C	═══	dialog at monitor
4.3	generating	G	≡≡≡	create program
4.4	controlling	T	------------	start program
5	page	F	⬭	overall system subsystem program

Table 4.1 Means of description in DRS

Persons. Because of their features, persons are at once static and dynamic elements, with the limitation that they are always elementary. They are termed homogeneous if they stand for a type; they can then be described more closely by their features in the descriptive part. In the survey they are listed by activity. Different types can be grouped as heterogeneous persons and further differentiated in the descriptive part.

Relations. Static and dynamic elements and persons can be related to each other by connecting lines. Relations are differentiated into the following groups: reading/writing, communicating, generating, and controlling. All dynamic elements and persons can read or write in connection with static elements. Persons can communicate with dynamic elements; this can amount to the reading and writing of information. Persons or dynamic elements can generate dynamic elements as well as control each other.

The Frame. The frame is the only structural item in the design and representation method presented here. It groups the entire system or its parts together and is thus a dynamic element itself, but its inner structure is visible. By employing the magnifying technique, every dynamic element can become a frame.

Table 4.2 contains an overview of how the individual elements of representation can be related to each other. Other linkage operations are not permitted in the DRS. Each of these tupels can be used to form complex structures if the operation is between two elements of the same kind. In addition, there are a number of rules:

R1: Reading access is always from the top; writing access is always to the bottom.
The controlling relation is directed from the top to the bottom. Communication is either undirected, and is then recorded horizontally, or it is directed. In the latter case, the higher element begins the communication.

R2: Static elements outside the frame are permanently at the level considered, while static elements within the frame are temporarily at the level considered.

R3: Temporal connections are given by the position of a dynamic element within a frame. Elements further to the top occur earlier, those to the bottom later.

R4: Every dynamic element may appear only once within a frame.

R5: Every static element may occur either exactly one time within a frame or exactly one time above and/or below a frame.

R6: A static element can only appear at the elementary level of description if it originated at a higher level of abstraction or earlier in time, is the object of writing and reading at the same level, or is created by the user.

R7: The designation for the level of abstraction is located in the upper left corner and begins with **A** for the system overview. The dynamic elements and persons within a frame are numbered with Arabic numerals. At the next lower level of abstraction the letter and number of the specified dynamic element are given at the lower right edge of the frame. This procedure is repeated down to the elementary descriptive level.

R8: Static elements are labelled if they are elementary. They are given a definite name, that is, maintained in the descriptive part.

R9: At the elementary level of description the design is structured so that dynamic elements appear only after a person; this applies to all frames in which persons appear.

In addition to these rules, which must be strictly observed, it is advisable for the sake of a design's clarity to order the elements so that the connecting lines do not cross and to put static elements appearing both above and below the frame into the same column if possible.

Description

The descriptive part is the verbal component of the DRS. Forms are used here as far as possible. For the statics of the design these are the data sheets, for the dynamics the algorithm sheets and the descriptions of activity. The description of the user interface is given as far as possible by state transition diagrams (see JACOB 1983). Where part structures can be executed in addition to the maximal precedence structures which can be recognized in the graphic representation, the part structures are also entered on a precedence table. The DRS components

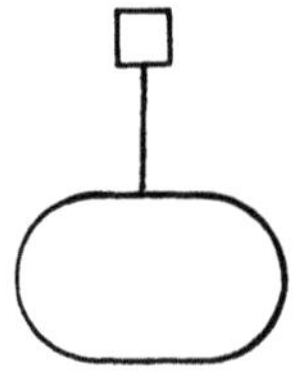	DE writes according to SE	printout of a list
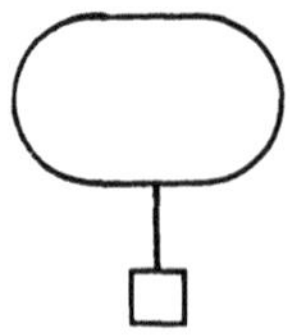	DE reads out of SE	read data set
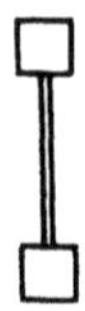	DE communicates with DE	
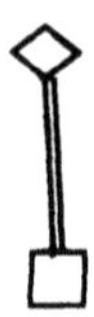	P communicates with DE	dialog with monitor
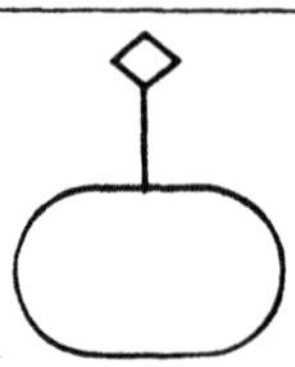	P writes according to SE	filling out a questionair
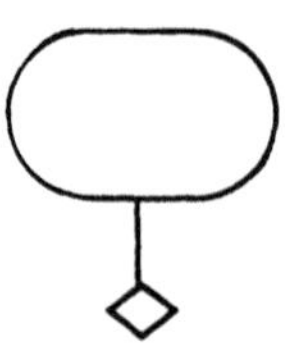	P reads out of SE	read computer printout

Table 4.2 Permissible links between means of representation

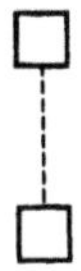	1 2	DE 2 is triggered automatically
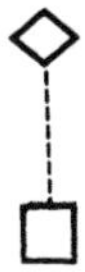		DE is triggered manually start program
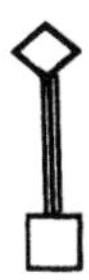		DE is created and triggered manually
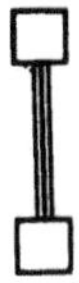	1 2	DE 2 is created and triggered automatically
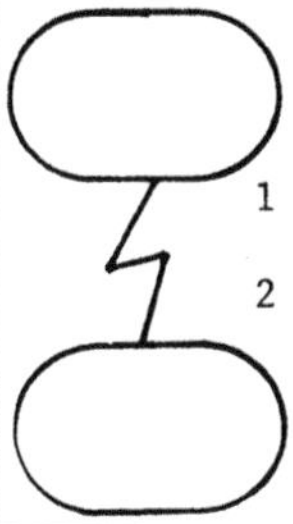	1 2	long-distance data transfer from SE1 to SE2

Table 4.2 continued

are listed again in Table 4.3.

REPRESENTATION PART graphic	general	state-function diagram
	fine	structogram
DESCRIPTIVE PART verbal	static	data sheets
	dynamic	algorithm sheets description of activity
	precedence	precedence graph

Table 4.3 Overview of DRS

The DRS system environment is now put over the system design achieved with the DRS as the highest level of abstraction, which is the same for all designs. The environment consists of three dynamic elements: the **monitor**, the **system activities**, and the **software tools**. The task of the monitor is to process and control the precedence structures of the individual system activities in the design. The software tools ensure the ability to keep the system flexible and to adjust it to later changes and extensions. The only static element at this level is the area of communications, which represents the interface between monitor and system activities.

Computer Aid for DRS

DRS is conceived so that the entire design can be prepared interactively at a graphic visual data unit connected with a plotter (in preparation; the design of the TBS was simulated by hand since the technical capacity available to the author in Ulm has so far not permitted the development of such a tool). The observance of the design rules is supervised, and planning aids are available. Moreover, the DRS derives the appropriate precedence graphs from the graphic representation; this graph can directly enter the generating at the monitor. Also, the static elements can be submitted to a test of plausibility and consistency. Three DRS types can be distinguished on the basis of their sequence in the overall design:

- Data sources: static elements which are read only.
- Data storage units: static elements which are both read and described. They are to be initiated at system implementation if they are to be read first, given that the precedences are observed.
- Data sinks: static elements which are described only.

The system designer can use these distinctions to check the consistency of his design.

Theoretical Foundation
The descriptive elements of DRS can be traced back to levels and channels, thus making it possible to describe the DRS with Petri nets.

General Design Rules
The following comments are intended to assist the system designer to prepare a design which will also suit the user:

- Feedback: The user should always be able to recognize the system's state, and the different system states should also be clearly distinguished.

- Similarity between command sequences and system answers: Different classes of system performance should also have clearly different appearances.

- System activities should be as reversible as possible: Where this is not possible and grave consequences might therefore result, the access to such activities should be limited.

- Consistency: The system should be consistent with regard to command structure and form.

- Error messages: User errors should be exactly localized in the input text. The context, descriptions of errors, and correction aids should be available. Error messages and their handling should be conducted at a special module.

- Aid functions: Only simple aid functions should be made available. More pdetailed user aid should be available in the form of written documentation.

4.2.3 Comments on Software Ergonomics

Ergonomics, the science of a worker's possible performance and limits and of the best possible mutual adjustment of man and his working conditions, first came into contact with information science via the industrial design of video workstations. Hardware ergonomics has by now become an everyday term as a result of extensive marketing by computer companies. Software ergonomics, in contrast, is new, and is not contained in many dictionaries of data processing terminology.

GRIESE (1982) defines software ergonomics as "adjusting software to man", distinguishing also between the creation of software and its use. In a larger framework, software ergonomics was a topic for the first time at last year's conference of the German chapter of the ACM in Nuremberg. There, in addition to established knowledge on, for example, the psychology of perception (MORITZ 1983) and the criteria for software design based on psychology and the study of work (RÖDIGER and NULLMEIER 1983), the "baby shoes" of the discipline were very apparent. Slogans such as "The aim is not a computer-oriented man, but the man-oriented computer"! (BALZERT 1983, p.15) can truly create the impression that "the power of the computers and the impotence of reason" is the out-moded view of an outsider (WEIZENBAUM 1977). A thesis such as "The user interface in a computer system is more than an auxiliary component; it must be tightly connected with all the components of a system and should be the starting point of the design process" (FISCHER 1983) may even support this impression, although it is hardly more than a platitude from the viewpoint of software development methodology (see Sect. 4.2.2). Leafing further through the conference reports, however, ample opportunity is provided to refute this view. The "compulsive programmer" hit more than one (WEIZENBAUM 1976). There we can find masks, apparently intended for German data inputers, that are interspersed with English commentaries and command words (HERCZEG 1983, p. 138), and others in which superimposed windows celebrate their virginal condition (PILLER 1983, p. 224). It is just too apparent: the computer has not lost its magical powers. Software ergonomists stare, as if under a spell, at the "peephole" called a screen, as if it were a master key to ergonomics. They do not notice that they attempt to attract people to the machine by means of more and more clever visual stimuli and thus achieve exactly what they actually wanted to avoid: man orients himself again according to the computer. In practice it is sufficient to convince management of the computer's newest tricks. The actual user is generally not asked, at the most, tested (e.g., BENDA 1983; LÜKE 1983). Especially ludicrous traits are shown by the development of the newest ergonomics hit, the touch-on screen, which treats the user completely as if he were an infant and lets him play on the screen with his fingers. It does not take much imagination to remember the experiments behavioralists conducted with apes in a similar way in order to determine whether the apes posses intelligence, and if so, how much. It seems as if it were high time to deal with questions of ethics rather than with questions of ergonomics. However that may be, there is still a long distance to "cognitive engineering", as NORMAN (1983, p. 257) suggests. To make a start at all, he recommends three methodological orientations:

1. Psychological mechanisms
2. User models
3. Analysis of user behavior

The development ot the TBS was oriented around these three points. Another principle that was followed was to keep the number and size of the man-machine interfaces as small as possible. (For a critical evaluation of the concepts of man-machine interface and man-machine communication see NAKE 1983). The advantages of the computer lie in the new possibilities that it creates and not in a person's occupation with the machine itself.

The practical consequences include, for example, two aspects of the TBS system design, whose usefulness can be documented in the relevant literature. Turning first to the help functions, in the TBS the user is only able to get information about the state of the system at one level, namely information about how to continue the dialogue. Not offered are the help systems which are being incorporated in more and more systems, and which either offer information on many different levels or even make the entire documentation available on-line. The reasons for this limitation in the TBS are that it is considered psychologically better for the user not to be deprived of all haptic qualities, such as handling and leafing in a documentation, when working with a computer, and that the system thus stays "handier". Furthermore, the system retains its topological qualities. Finally, one last reason was revealed in a study by DUNSMORE (1980), who confirmed in experiments that people who use a written documentation show better performance than those who only have an on-line documentation at their disposal.

The other example refers to the correction of incorrect or unknown word forms. In these cases a manual/intellectual step is intentionally used in the TBS; however, this step is computer aided in that the computer prints a so-called red printout, on which the incorrect and unknown word forms are in red in contrast to the rest of the text printed in black. In the dialogue with the TBS only the red word forms are displayed and the user makes a decision based on his printout. This approach is given support by a study by WRIGHT and LICKORISH (1983); in an experiment they demonstrated not only that incorrect word forms are detected more rapidly in a printed text but that nearly all mistakes are detected there. In contrast, test persons detected significantly fewer mistakes at a visual display unit, and even required more time.

The book by GILB and WEINBERG (1977) was taken as a guide for the general structure of the man-machine dialogue in the TBS. Although already 8 years old, measured by the ideas it contains it is still young and suited for modern tasks. The quality of this book is also very apparent in its typographical form and didactic structure.

4.3 Creating the TBS

The architecture of the TBS is presented in this section in the form it was developed, using the DRS as design methodology, and then actually created on the TR440, as far as technically possible. In order to keep the size of the description within limits, not all nonelementary dynamic elements are followed to the elementary level. They are labeled with an X in the graphs (e.g., for A1B1 "recode"). A more detailed verbal description has already been given in Sect. 2.4.

Two tables follow the representation part. The first gives a survey of the static elements contained in the design in relation to the dynamic elements working with them. The data collections can be classified using this information because of the time relations given in the DRS (it follows, for example, that dynamic elements with smaller numbers take place earlier). The data collection sheets are pure input data because they are only read; they are always provided to the system from the outside. In contrast, the pseudonym storage unit is first read and later also described. This file must be initiated at the system implementation. An example of a temporary file is a concordance of pseudonyms, which is only required for the manual distribution of pseudonyms.

This last table gives the precedences which can be derived from the graphic representation. Sequentially occurring processes are listed below each other, those in parallel next to each other. The bold face numbers stand for dynamic elements in which persons are active first. For the monitor this means a break in the automatically controlled operations, transferring the decision to the user or administrator. In the current form of the TBS, these blocks (see the tables) take the form of procedures which create an job for each element and insert it in the batch of jobs waiting to be processed. This cascade principle has made it possible for several users to use the text base simultaneously (each virtually with a text base of their own) despite the limitations imposed by the TR440.

The replacement of the TR440 by two systems of the next generation (Siemens 7550 under BS2000; VAX 8600 under VMS) which has now begun means that the technical prerequisites are being created for achieving the potential still contained in the TBS design. This will make it possible for the cascade operation to be replaced in part by a partner operation. User guidance will then proceed by means of masks and menus, as described in Chap. 2.

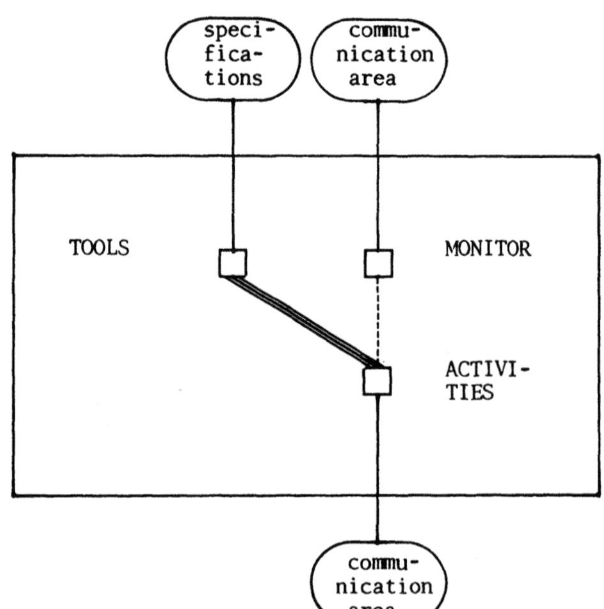
speci-
fica-
tions
commu-
nication
area
TOOLS
MONITOR
ACTIVI-
TIES
commu-
nication
area

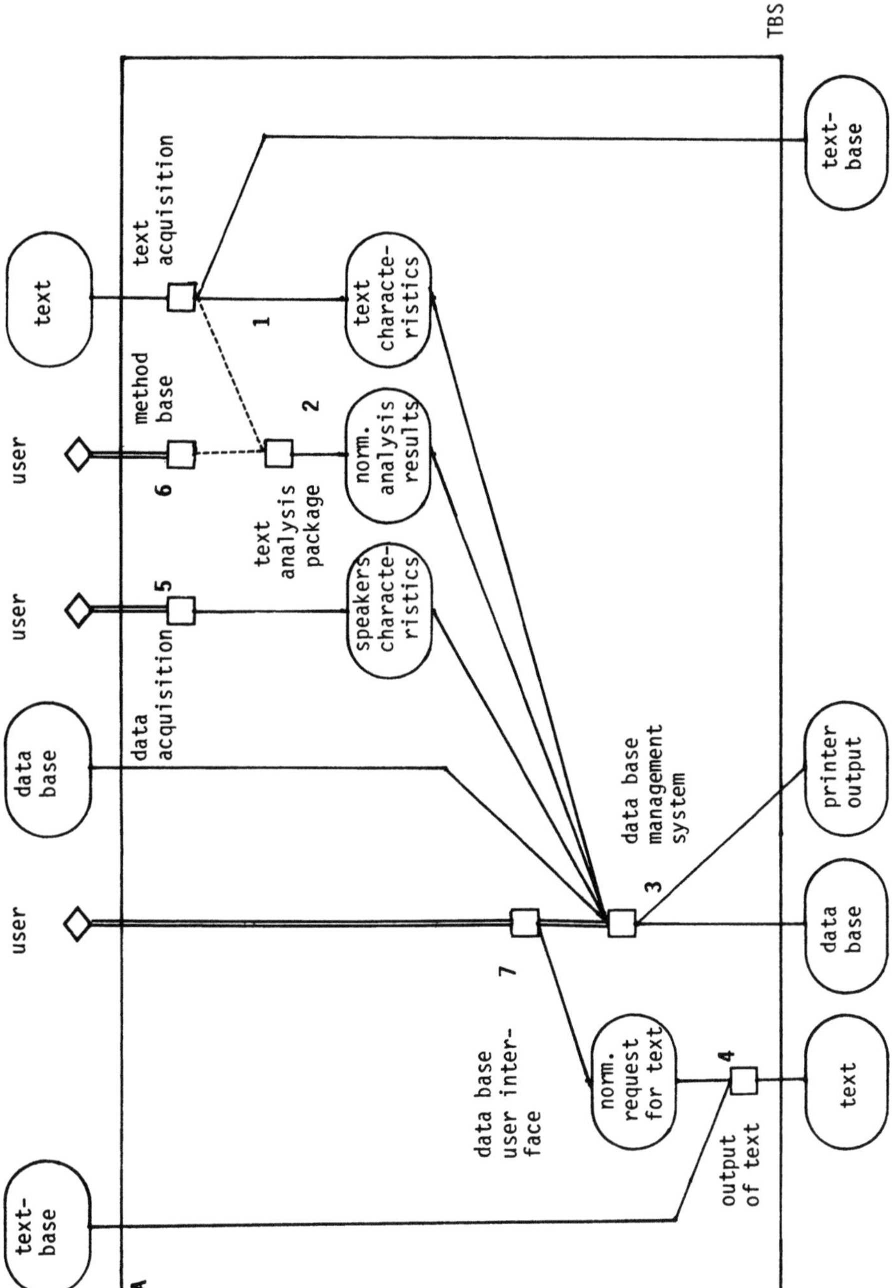

TBS
A
text
user
user
data base
user
text-base
text acquisition
method base
data acquisition
1
2
5
6
text analysis package
text characte- ristics
norm. analysis results
speakers characte- ristics
data base management system
3
7
4
data base user inter- face
norm. request for text
output of text
text- base
printer output
data base
text

ACQUISITION OF TEXT

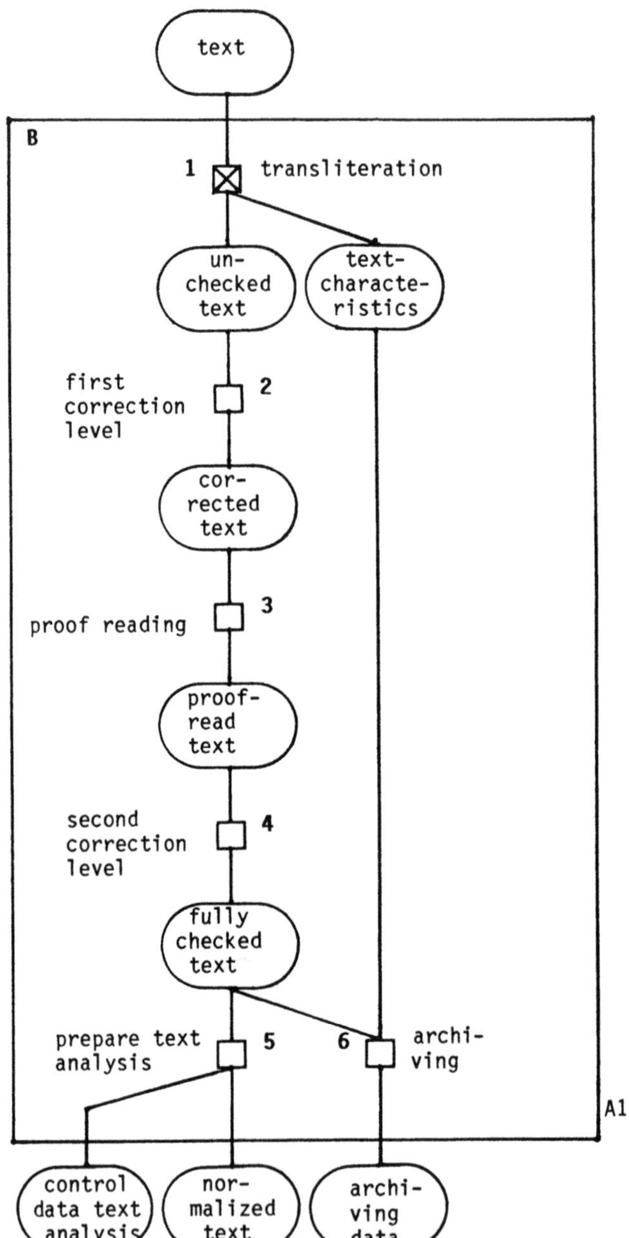

FIRST CORRECTION LEVEL

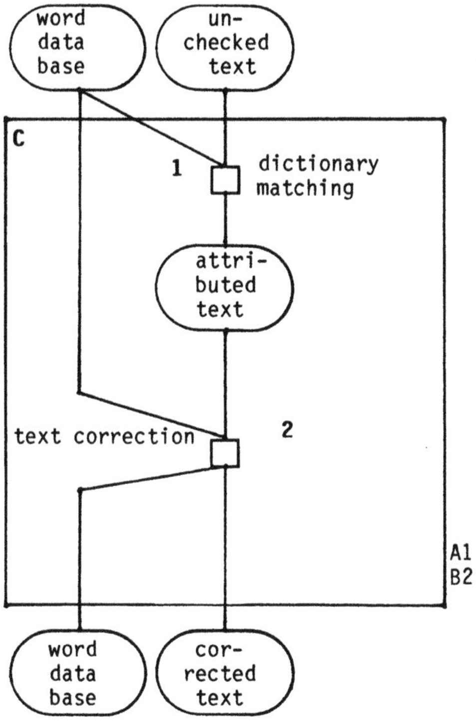

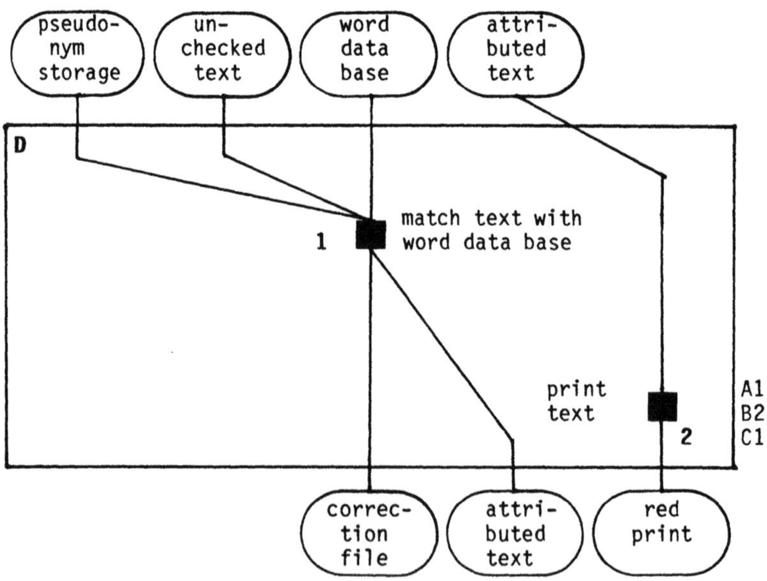
pseudo-
nym
storage
un-
checked
text
word
data
base
attri-
buted
text
D
match text with
word data base
1
print
text
2
A1
B2
C1
correc-
tion
file
attri-
buted
text
red
print

TEXT CORRECTION

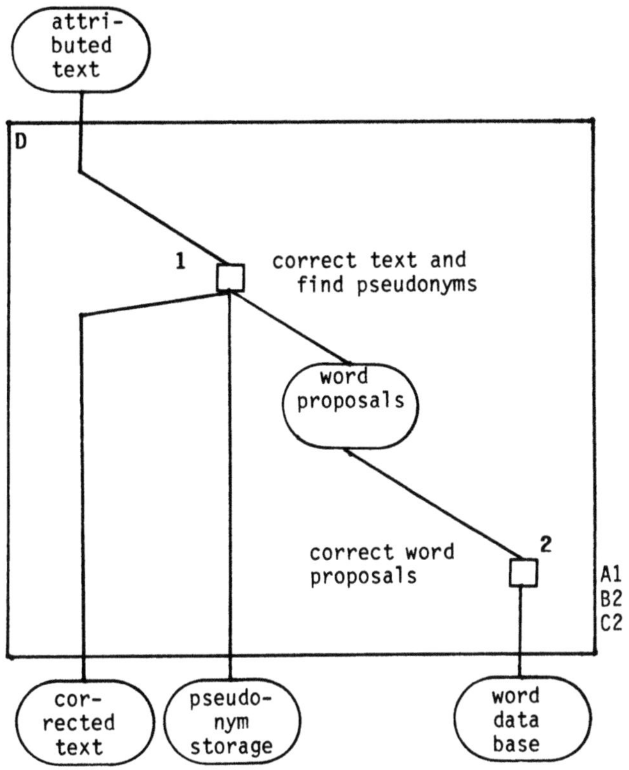

CORRECT TEXT AND FIND PSEUDONYMS

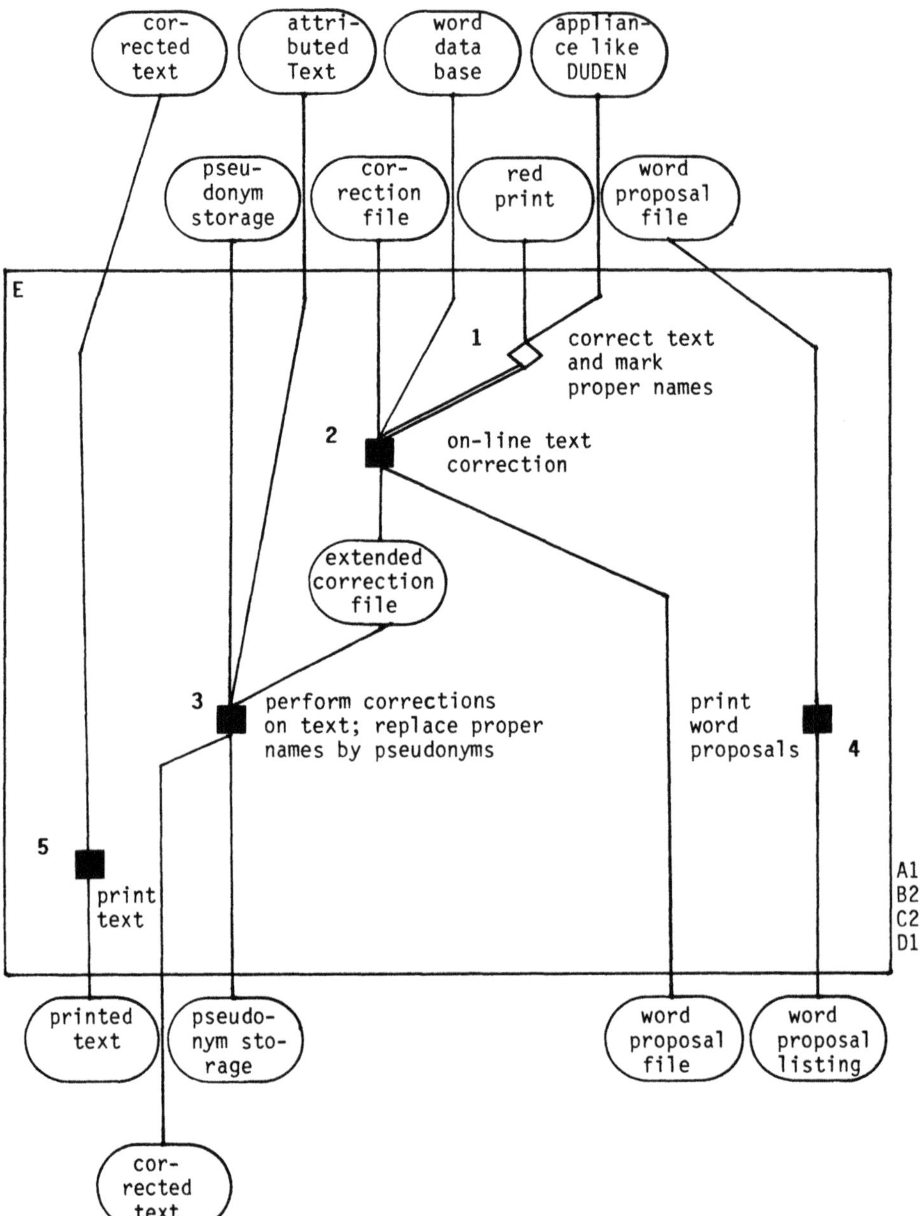

CORRECT WORD PROPOSALS

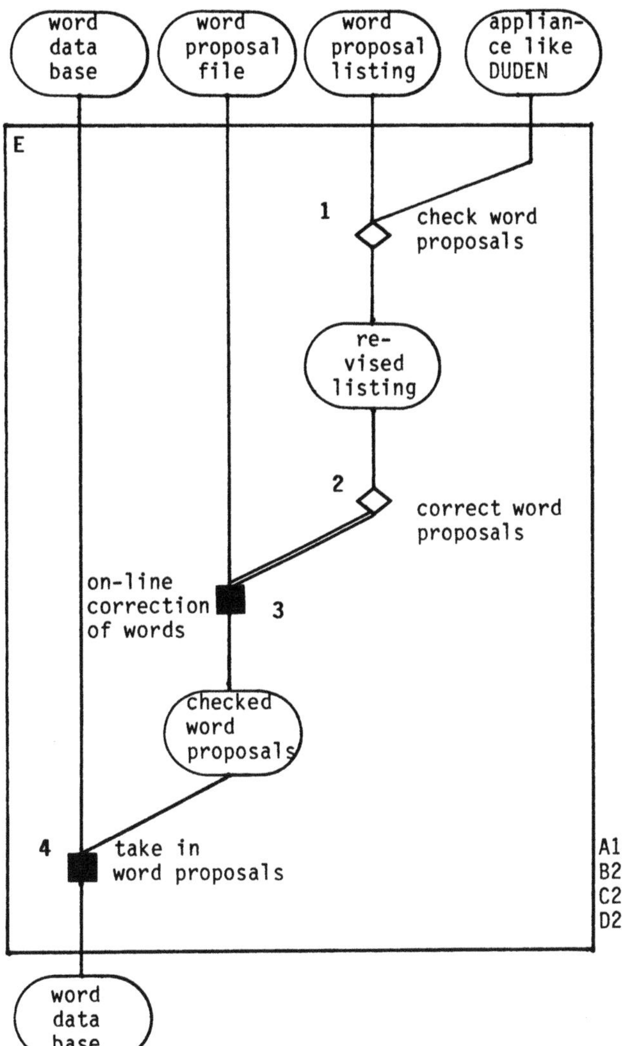

PROOF READING

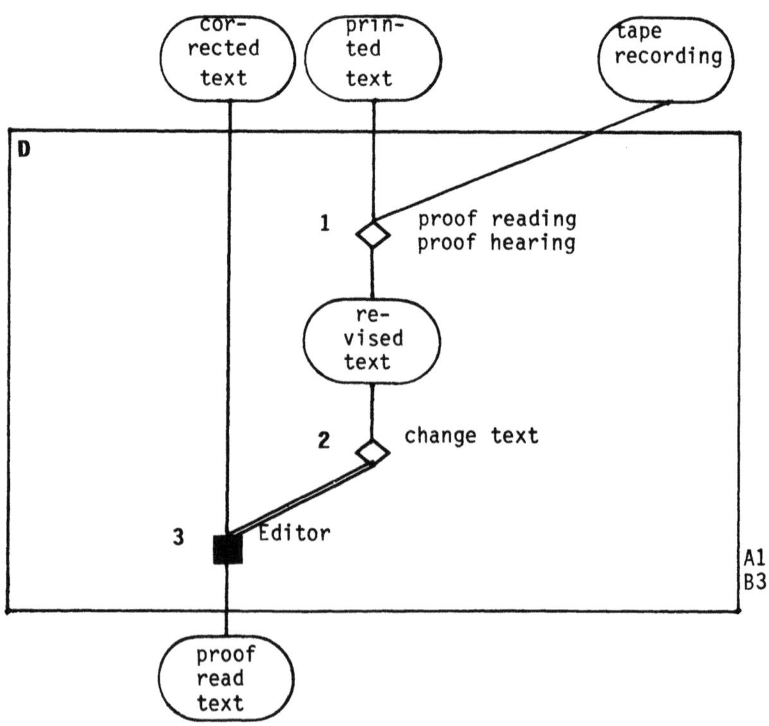

SECOND CORRECTION LEVEL

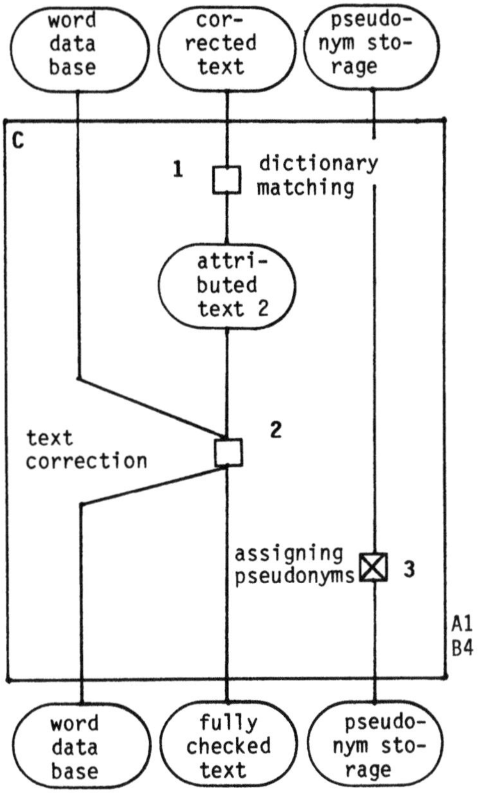

SECOND DICTIONARY MATCHING

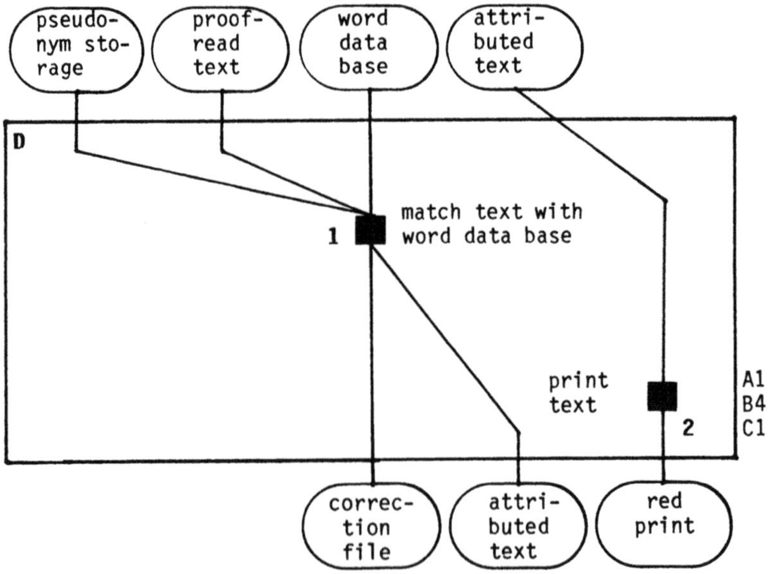

SECOND TEXT CORRECTION

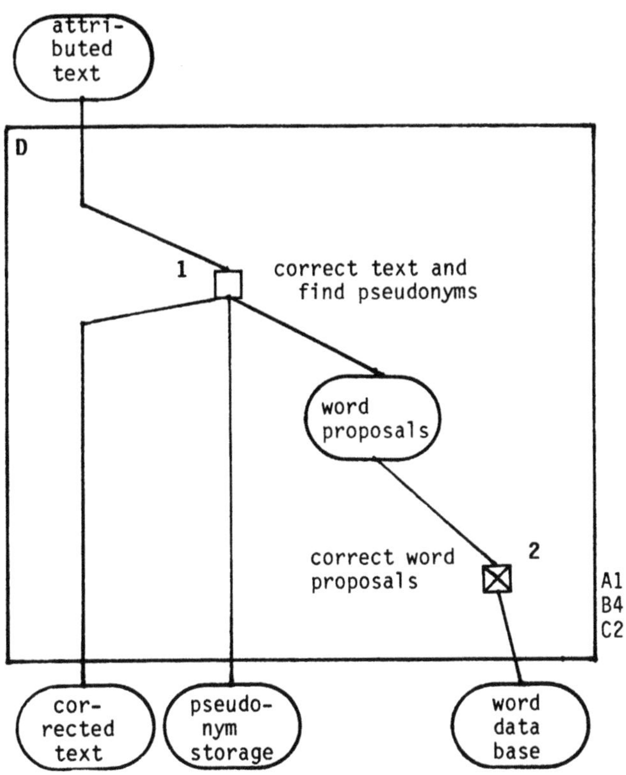

CORRECT TEXT AND FIND PSEUDONYMS

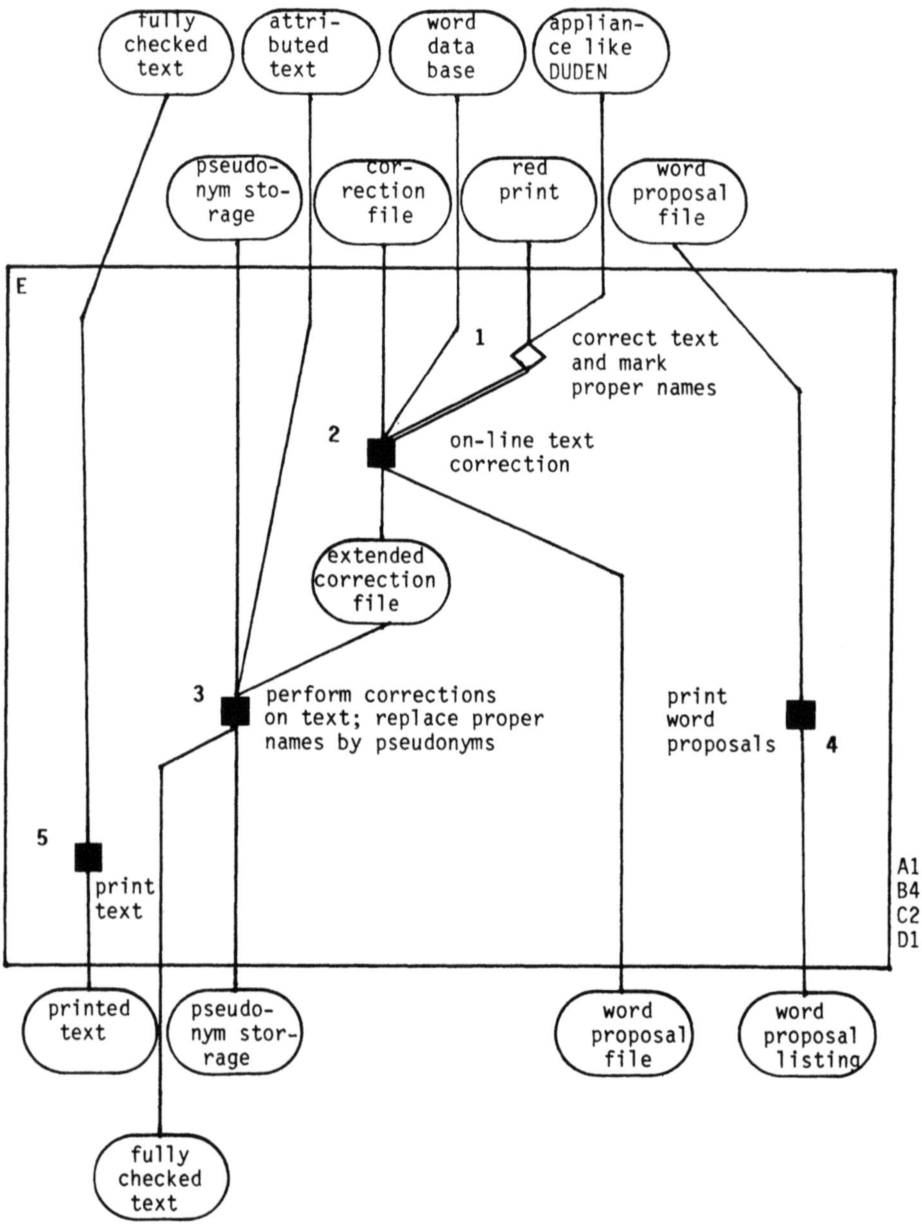

ASSIGNING PSEUDONYMS

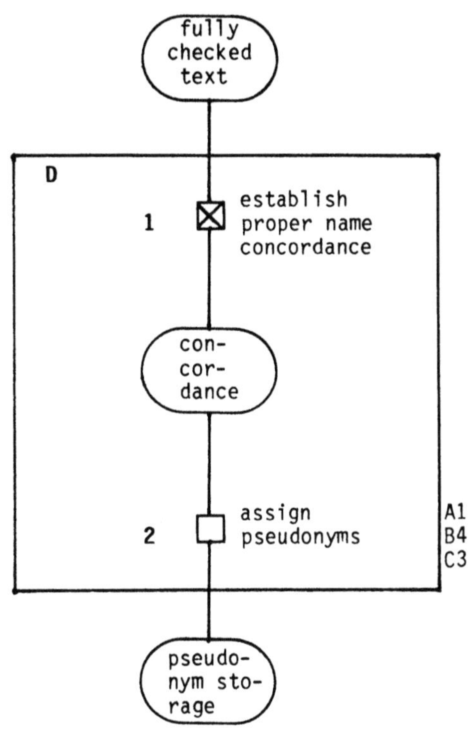

ASSIGN PSEUDONYMS

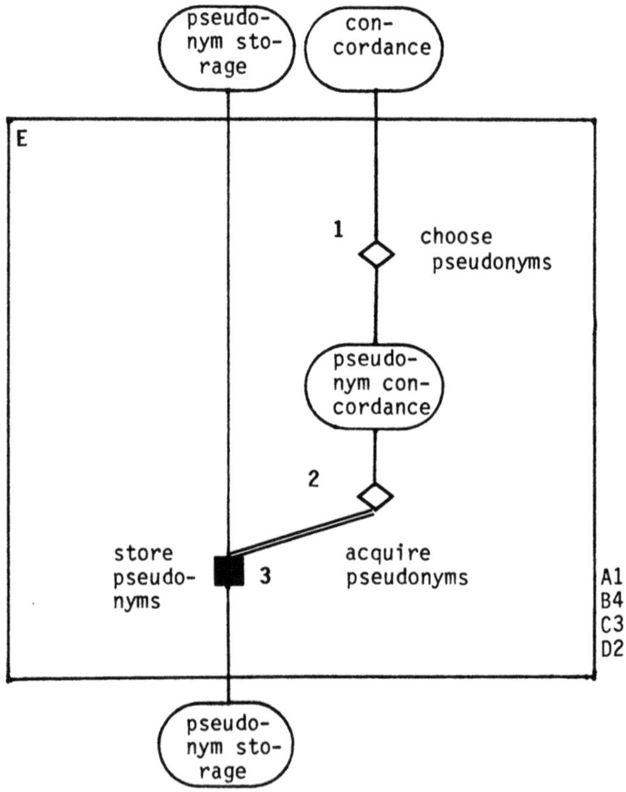

PREPARE TEXTANALYSIS

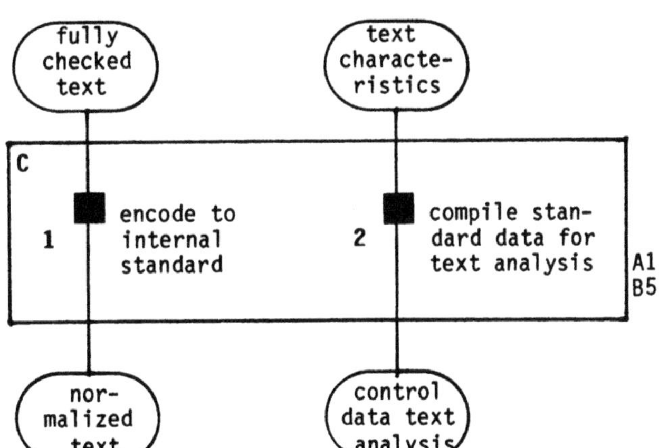

ARCHIVING

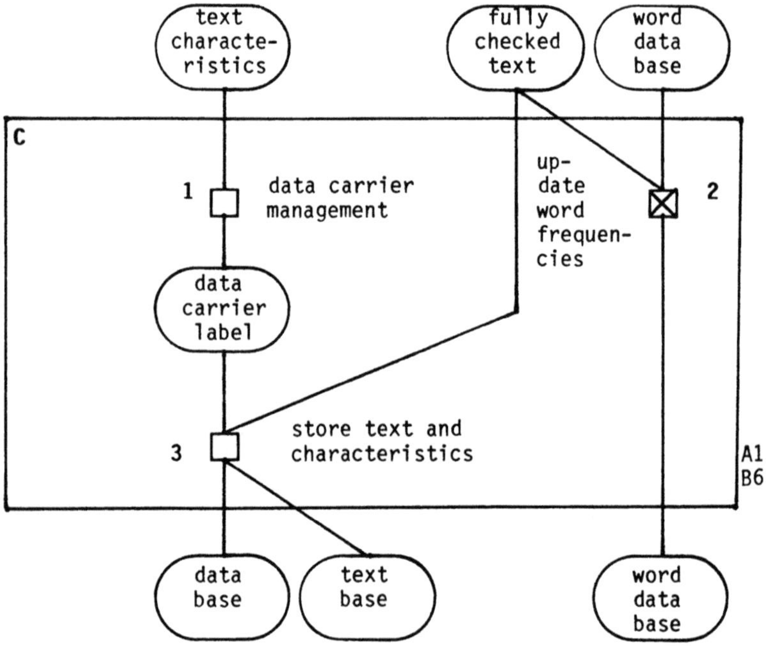
text characte- ristics
fully checked text
word data base
C
1
data carrier management
up- date word frequen- cies
2
data carrier label
3
store text and characteristics
A1
B6
data base
text base
word data base

DATA CARRIER MANAGEMENT

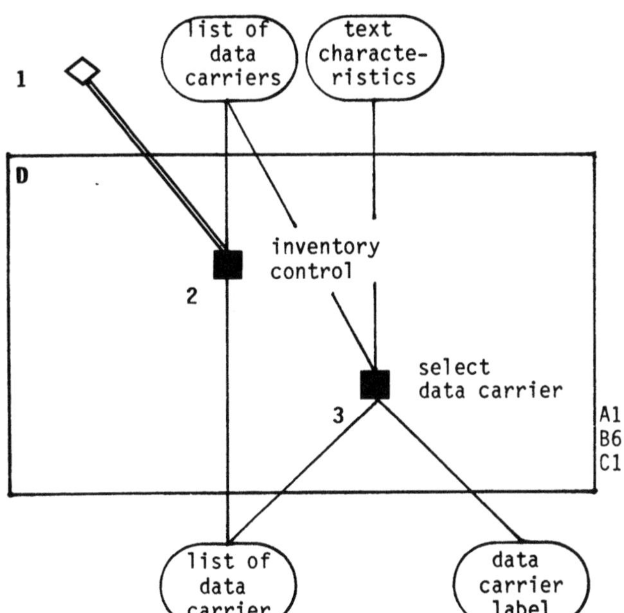

STORE TEXT AND CHARACTERISTICS

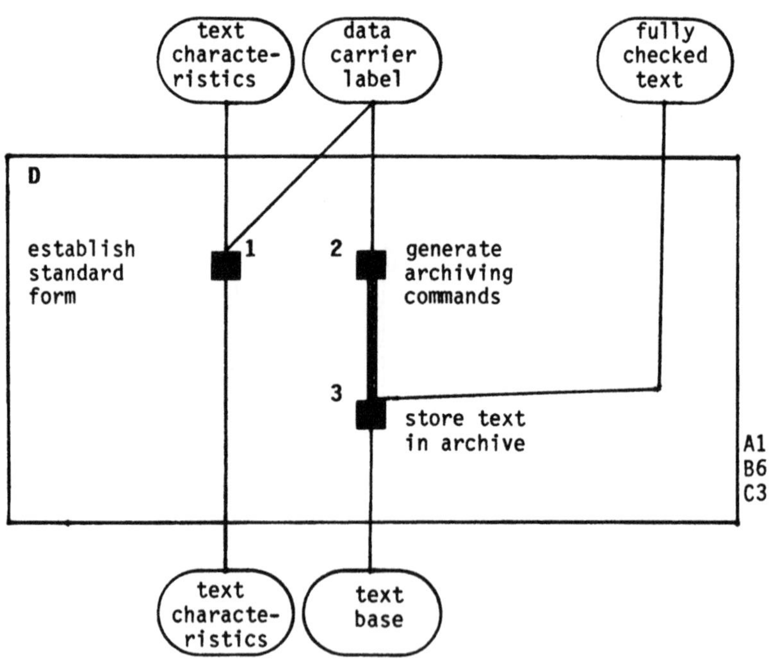

TEXT ANALYSIS

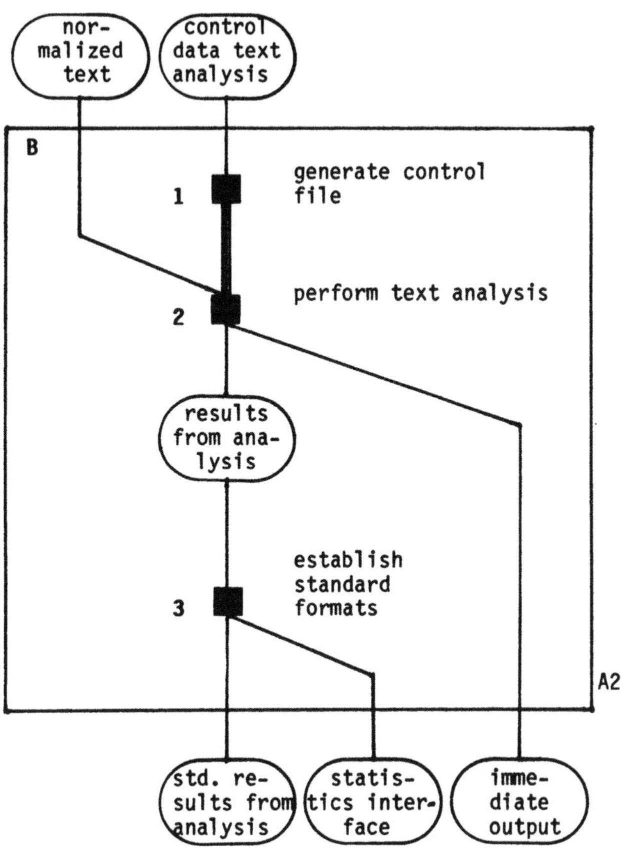

DATA BASE MANAGEMENT SYSTEM

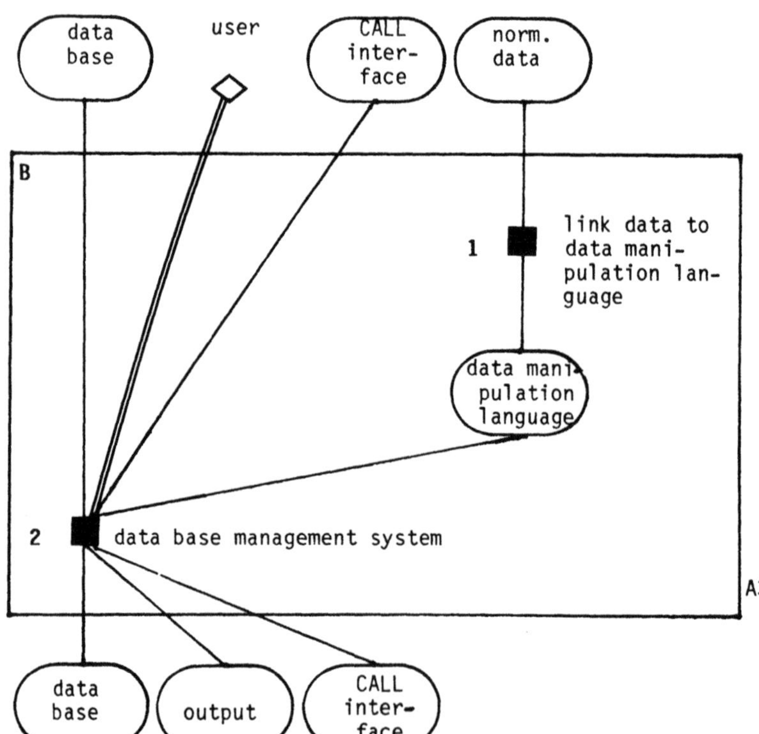

TEXT OUTPUT

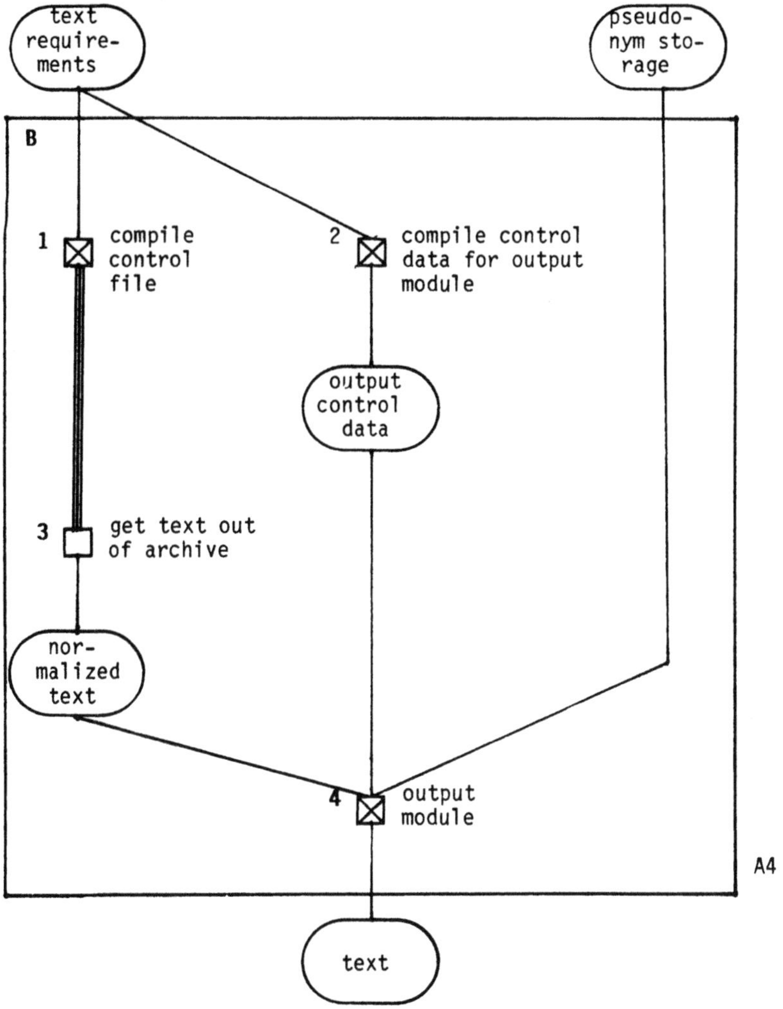
text requirements
pseudonym storage
B
1
compile control file
2
compile control data for output module
output control data
3
get text out of archive
normalized text
4
output module
A4
text

GET TEXT OUT OF ARCHIVE

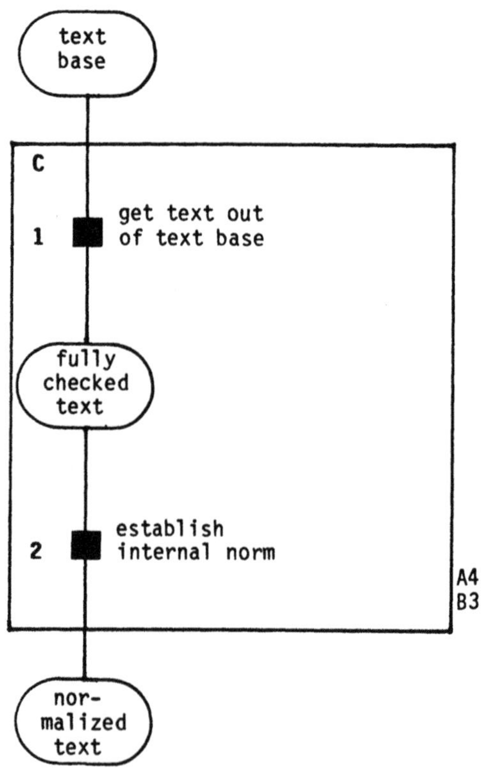

ACQUIRE CHARACTERISTIC DATA

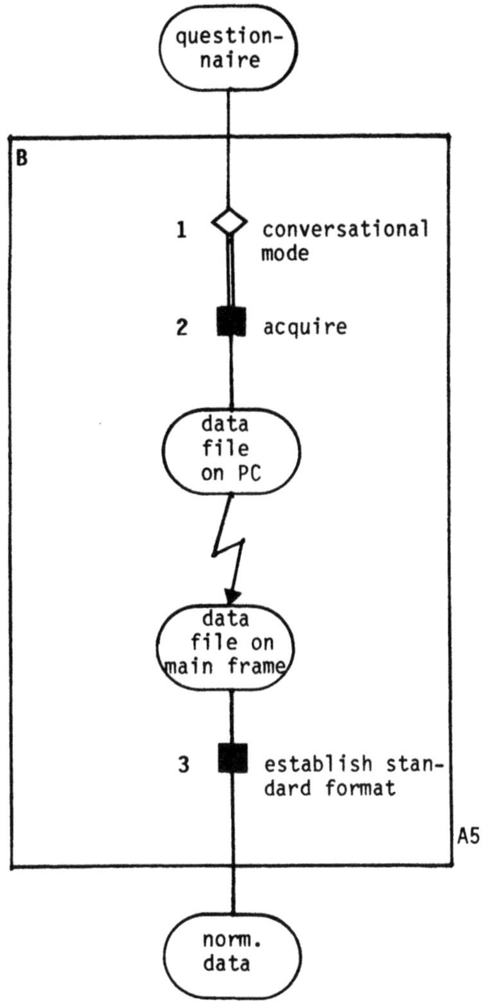

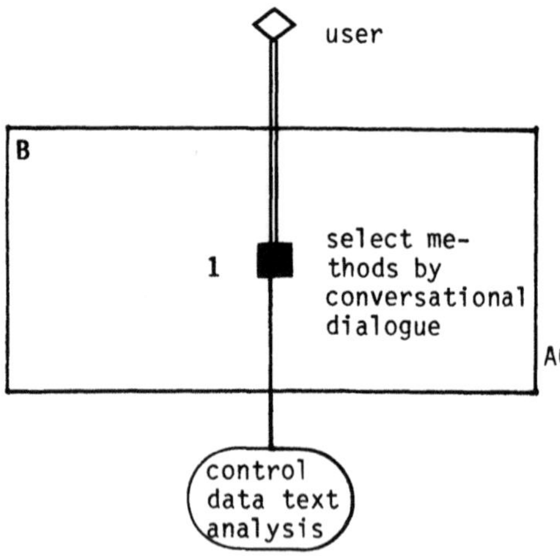
user
B
1
select methods by conversational dialogue
A6
control data text analysis

USER MODULE

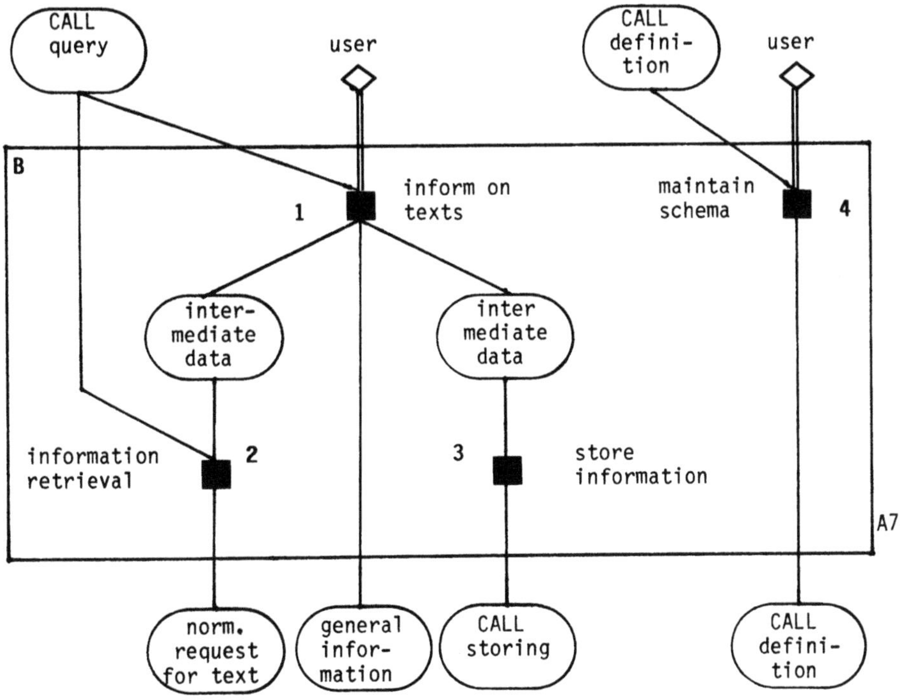
CALL query
user
CALL definition
user
B
1
inform on texts
maintain schema
4
intermediate data
inter mediate data
information retrieval
2
3
store information
A7
norm. request for text
general information
CALL storing
CALL definition

ABCDE	ABCDE	ABCDE	ABCDE	ABCDE
11				
1211				
1212				
12211				
12212				
12213	12214			
12215				
12221				
12222				
12223				
12224				
1231				
12321				
12322				
12323				
131				
132				
133				
151	152	**1611**		
		1612	1613	162
		1631	1632	
			1633	
21				
22				
23				
31		31		
32		32		

Table 4.4 Precedence structures in TBS

References

Alekseev, P.M.: Statistische Lexikographie. Zur Typologie, Erstellung und Anwendung von Frequenzwörterbüchern. Studienverlag Dr. N. Brockmeyer, Bochum 1984.

Altmann, G.: Towards a Theory of Language. In: Altmann, G. (Ed.): Glottometrika 1: 1-25, Studienverlag Dr. N. Brockmeyer, Bochum 1978.

Altmann, G. und Kind, B.: Ein semantisches Gesetz. In: Köhler, R. und Boy, J.: Glottometrika 5: 1-13, Studienverlag Dr. N. Brockmeyer, Bochum 1982.

Aphek, E. and Tobin, Y.: Word Systems and the Language of Family Therapy. 12. Weltkongreß für Soziologie, Mexiko 1982.

Bänninger-Huber, E.: Die Anwendung von FACS zur Evaluation eines neuen Therapiekonzepts für Stotterer. In: Bänninger-Huber, E., Schneider, H. und Steiner, F. (Hrsg.): Nonverbales Verhalten als Indikator für kognitiv-affektive Prozesse in der Psychotherapie. Berichte Nr. 17 des Psychologischen Instituts der Universität Zürich 1984.

Balzert, H. (Hg.): Software-Ergonomie. Tagung des German Chapter of the ACM in Nürnberg 1983. Teubner, Stuttgart 1983.

Basili, V.R. and Perricone, B.T.: Software Errors and Complexity: An Empirical Investigation. Communications of the ACM 27(1): 42-52 (1984).

Bausch, K.-H.: Zur Umschrift gesprochener Hochsprache. In: Steger, H. (Hg.): Texte gesprochener deutscher Standardsprache I: 33-54, Institut für deutsche Sprache, Freiburg 1971.

Beermann, S.: Linguistische Analyse psychoanalytischer Therapiedialoge unter besonderer Berücksichtigung passiver Sprechmuster. Staatsexamensarbeit, Universität Hamburg 1983.

Benda, von H.: Feldversuch zur Gestaltung des Mensch-Maschine-Dialogs. In: Balzert, H. (Hg.): Software-Ergonomie. German Chapter of the ACM Berichte Bd. 14: 266-277, Teubner, Stuttgart 1983.

Bennett, W.R.: How Artificial is Intelligence? American Scientist 65: 694-702 (1977).

Bergmann und Henning: Lemmatisierung in HAM-ANS. Forschungsstelle für Informationswissenschaft und Künstliche Intelligenz. Universität Hamburg 1982.

Blanck, J. and Krijger, M.J. (Eds.): Methods and Techniques in Software Engineering. Wiley, New York 1983.

Boder, D.P.: The Adjective-Verb-Quotient: A Contribution to the Psychology of Language. In: Psychological Record 3: 310-343 (1940).

Bodmer, W.: Quantifizierbare Aspekte von Dialogen - Ihre Operationalisierung und deren Interpretation auf werk- und textsortenspezifischer Ebene. Lizentiatsarbeit an der Universität Zürich 1981.

Böckmann, H.-G.: Ergänzungen bei Struktogrammen. Angewandte Informatik 8: 330-336 (1983).

Böhm, C. and Jacopini, G.: Flow Diagrams, Turing Machines and Languages with only two Formation Rules. Commun. ACM 9: 366-371 (1966).

Boot, M.: Linguistic Data Structure. Reducing Encoding by Hand and Programming Languages. In: Jones, A.J. and Churchhouse, R.F. (Eds.): The Computer in Literary and Linguistic Studies. 255-270, University of Wales Press, Cardiff 1976.

Boot, M.: An Experimental Design for Automatic Syntactic Encoding of Natural Language Texts. ALLC-Bulletin 5: 237-241 (1977).

Boot, M.: Homographie. Ein Beitrag zur automatischen Wortklassenzuweisung in der Computerlinguistik. Unveröffentlichte Dissertation Utrecht 1978.

Brähler, E.: Die Erfassung des Interventionsstils von Therapeuten durch die automatische Sprachanalyse. Zeitschrift für Psychosomatische Medizin und Psychoanalyse 24: 156-168 (1978).

Brähler, E., und Zenz, H.: Apparative Analyse des Sprechverhaltens in der Psychotherapie. Zeitschrift für Psychosomatische Medizin und Psychoanalyse 20(4): 328-336 (1974).

Brunner, E.J. und Mergenthaler, E.: Erfassung von Kommunikationsmustern in Familien über die Analyse von Sprecherabfolgen. Vortrag, gehalten auf der 23. Tagung der experimentell arbeitenden Psychologen, Berlin 1981.

Brustkern, J. and Schulze, W.: Towards a Cumulated Word Data Base for the German Language. IKP-Arbeitsberichte Nr. 1: 1-9, Universität Bonn 1983.

Brustkern, J., Schlimgen, E. and Schulze, W.: Selected Bibliography on Machine-Readable Dictionaries. IKP-Arbeitsberichte Nr. 1. Universität Bonn 1983.

Brustkern, J., Heinze, G. und Schulze, W.: Die Wortdatenbank des Deutschen. Vortrag am Institut für deutsche Sprache, Mannheim 1984.

Burner, S.: Delire Clos et Delire Ouvert. ALLC Journal 12(1): 19 (1984).

Busemann, A.: Die Sprache der Jugend als Ausdruck der Entwicklungsrhythmik. Jena 1925.

Calzolari, N.: Lexical Definitions in a Computerized Dictionary. Computers & Artificial Intelligence 2: 225-233 (1983).

Chomsky, N.: Aspects of the Theory of Syntax. MIT-Press, Cambridge/Mass 1965. In Deutsch: Aspekte der Syntax Theorie. Suhrkamp, Frankfurt 1965.

Cierpka, M.: Personalpronomina als Indikatoren für interpersonale Beziehungen in einer psychoanalytischen Gruppentherapie. Med. Diss. Universität Ulm 1978.

Clippinger, J.: A Discourse Speaking Program as a Preliminary Theory of Discourse Behavior and a Limited Theory of Psychoanalytic Discourse. University Microfilms International Ann Arbor, Michigan USA 1974.

Codd, E.F.: A Relational Model of Data for Large Shared Data Banks.

Communications of the ACM 13(6): 377-387 (1970).

COMPACT (Computergestütztes Programmier- (Problemlösungs-) Unterstützungssystem Actis). Fa. Actis GmbH, Stuttgart.

Cremerius, J.: Schweigen als Problem der psychoanalytischen Technik. Jahrbuch der Psychoanalyse 6: 69-103 (1969).

Croft, W.B. and Pezarro, M.T.: Text Retrieval Techniques for the Automated Office. In: Naffah, N. (Ed.): Office Information Systems. Proceedings of the 2nd. International Workshop on Office Information Systems, Oct. 1981. North-Holland, Amsterdam 1982.

Dagwell, R. and Weber, R.: System Designers' User Models: A Comparative Study and Methodological Critique. Communications of the ACM 26(11): 987-997 (1983).

Dahl, H.: Word Frequency of Spoken American English. Verbatim, Essex Conn. 1979.

Daniels, H.-J.: Die Bedeutung des Pflichtenheftes für den Software-Entwicklungsprozeß. Angewandte Informatik 3: 87-97 (1984).

Dearnley, P.A. and Mayhew, P.J.: In Favour of System Prototypes and their Integration into the Systems Development Cycle. The Computer-Journal 26(1): 36-42 (1983).

Degenhardt, B. und Degenhardt, W.: SIR/DBMS in der qualitativen Forschung. ZUMA-Arbeitsbericht 84/01: 5-55, Mannheim 1984.

Dennins, J.B.: Betrieb von Rechensystemen, Begriffe, Auftragsabwicklung. Beuth, Berlin 1976.

Deutsch, F.: Analytic Posturology. Psychoanal. Quart. 21: 196-214 (1952).

Dijkstra, E.W.: A Construcitve Approach to the Problem of Program Correctness. BIT 8(3): 174-186 (1968a).

Dijkstra, E.W.: The Structure of the THE Multiprogramming System. Commun. ACM: 341-356 (1968b).

Dijkstra, E.W.: Goto Considered Harmful. Comm. ACM 11(3): 1968c

Dijkstra, E.W.: Structured Programming. In: Buxton, J.N. and Randell, B. (Eds.): Software Engineering Techniques: 88-93, NATO-Science-Committee, Brüssel 1970.

Dijkstra, E.W.: Notes on Structured Programming. Structured Programming, Academic Press, New York 1972.

Dietrich, R.: Automatische Textwörterbücher. Studien zur maschinellen Lemmatisierung verbaler Wortformen des Deutschen. Niemeyer, München 1972.

Drewek, R.: Einige formale Charakteristiken in Gesprächen mit mehreren Sprechern. Glottometrika 6: (1984).

Drewek, R. and Erni, M.: LDVLIB. A (new) Software Package for Text Research. Vortrag ALLC-Conference, Pisa 1982.

Duden: Das große Wörterbuch der deutschen Sprache in sechs Bänden. Bibliographisches Institut Mannheim 1976.

Duden Band 4: Grammatik der deutschen Gegenwartssprache. 3. Auflage. Bibliographisches Institut Mannheim 1973.

Duden Band 5: Fremdwörterbuch. 3. Auflage. Bibliographisches Institut Mannheim 1974.

Dürr, H.-G.: Die Integration der Textverarbeitung und schriftlichen Kommunikation in das Informationssystem des Unternehmens. In: GI-Fachtagung: Information Retrieval Systeme und Management Information Systeme, Vorabdruck der Vorträge, Stuttgart 1970.

Dunsmore, H.: Designing an Interactive Facility for Non-Programmers. Proceedings of the ACM 80: 475-483 (1980).

Eggeling, J.: GOTO - REPEAT UNTIL. Schwierigkeiten mit der Software. In: Michel, K.M. und Spengler T. (Hg.): Kursbuch 75. Computerkultur: 75-87, Rotbuch, Berlin 1984.

Ehlich, K. und Rehbein, J.: Halbinterpretative Arbeitstranskription (HIAT 1). Linguistische Berichte 45: 21-41 (1976).

Ehlich, K. und Rehbein, J.: Erweiterte halbinterpretative Arbeitstranskription (HIAT 2): Intonation. Linguistische Berichte 59: 51-75 (1979).

Eisenmann, F.: Die Satzkonjunktionen in gesprochener Sprache. Niemeyer, Tübingen, 1973.

Erben, J.: Deutsche Grammatik -ein Leitfaden-. Fischer, Frankfurt 1968.

Fährmann, R.: Die Deutung des Sprechausdrucks. Bouvier, Bonn 1967.

Fischer, G.: Entwurfsrichtlinien für die Software-Ergonomie aus der Sicht der Mensch-Maschine-Kommunikation (MMK). In: Balzert, H. (Hg.): Software-Ergonomie. German Chapter of the ACM Berichte Bd. 14.: 30-48, Teubner, Stuttgart 1983.

Flader, D. und Grodziki, W.-D.: Hypothesen zur Wirkungsweise der psychoanalytischen Grundregel. Psyche 32: 545-594 (1978).

Flader, D.: Die psychoanalytische Therapie als Gegenstand sprachwissenschaftlicher Forschung. Studium Linguistik 5: 23-36 (1978).

Flader, D. und Wodak-Leodolter, R. (Hg.): Therapeutische Kommunikation. Scriptor, Köngigstein/Ts. 1979.

Flader, D., Grodzicki, W.-D. und Schröter, K.: Psychoanalyse als Gespräch. Suhrkamp, Frankfurt 1982.

Flader, D. und Koerfer, A.: Die diskurslinguistische Erforschung von Therapiegesprächen. Osnabrücker Beiträge zur Sprachtheorie 24: 57-90 (1983).

Freud, S.: Schriften zur Behandlungstechnik. S.Fischer, Frankfurt/M. 1913.

Freud. S.: Vorlesung zur Einführung in die Psychoanalyse und Neue Folge. S.Fischer, Frankfurt/M. 1916/17.

Friedman, J.: A Computer System for Transformational Grammar. Communications of the ACM 12(6): 341-348 (1969).

Friedman, J. et al.: A Computer Model of Transformational Grammar. Elsevier, New York 1971.

Friedman, J.: Working with the Interactive Version of the Transformational Grammar tester of J.Friedman - International Conference on Computational Linguistics, Pisa 1973.

Gass, E., Gerne, M., Loepfe, M., Meier, B., Rothenfluh, Th. and Strauch, I.: Traumdatenbank (TDB). Manual für die standardisierte Gewinnung von Traumberichten im Labor und die Handhabung einer zugehörigen Datenbank auf dem Computer. Psychologisches Institut der Universität Zürich 1983.

Gerkens, R.M. und Winter, D.: ISAC - Die Einbettung der Methode in eine Software-Produktionsumgebung. Veröffentlichung Nr. 84/2 der Firma ACTIS, Stuttgart 1984.

Gersbach, B.: Die Vergangenheitstempora in oberdeutscher gesprochener Sprache. Niemeyer, Tübingen 1981.

Gilb, T. and Weinberg, G.M.: Humanized Input. Techniques for Reliable Keyed Input. Winthrop Publishers, Inc., Cambridge 1977.

Godbersen, H.P.: Funktionsnetze. Eine Modellierungskonzeption zur Entwurfs- und Entscheidungsunterstützung. Ladewig, München 1983.

Goeppert, S. und Goeppert, H.: Sprache und Psychoanalyse. Rowohlt, Reinbek 1973.

Gotthard, W., Zincke, G. und Dreckmann, K.-H.: ANIMOS - eine integrierte Methode zum Softwareentwurf. Angewandte Informatik 6: 225-233, 1984.

Gottschalk, L.A.: Quantificitaton and Psychological Indicators of Emotions: The Content Analysis of Speech and other Objective Measures of Psychological States. Int.J.Psychiatry in Medicine 5(4): 587-611 (1974).

Gottschalk, L.A.: The Psychoanalytic Study of Hand-Mouth Approximations. Psychoanalysis and Contemporary Science 3: 269-291 (1974).

Gottschalk, L.A. and Gleser, G.C.: The Measurement of Psychological States Through the Content Analysis of Verbal Behavior. Calif.Univ.-Press, Berkeley 1969.

Gottschalk, L.A. and Uliana, R.L.: Further Studies on the Relationship of non-verbal to verbal Behavior: Effect of Lip Caressing on Shame, Hostility, and Other Variables as Expressed in the Content of Speech. In: Freedman N. and Stanley G. (Eds.): Communicative Structures and Psychic Structures. 311-330, Plenum, New York 1977.

Griese, J.: Software Ergonomie. Informatik Spektrum 5(2): 124 (1982).

Gröben, N. und Westmeyer, H.: Kriterien psychologischer Forschung. Juventa, München 1975.

Grünzig, H.-J.: Zeitreihenanalyse psychoanalytischer Behandlungsverläufe: Stichprobenprobleme und erste Ergebnisse bei einem Einzelfall. In: Czogalik, D., Ehlers, W. und Teufel, R. (Hg.): Perspektiven der Psychotherapieforschung: Einzelfall-Gruppe-Institution. Hochschulverlag Freiburg 1984 (im Druck).

Grünzig, H.-J., Holzscheck, K. und Kächele, H.: EVA - Ein Programmsystem zur maschinellen Inhaltsanalyse von Psychotherapieprotokollen. Medizinische Psychologie 2: 208-217 (1976).

Grünzig, H.-J. und Mergenthaler, E.: Computerunterstützte Ansätze. Empirische Untersuchungen am Beispiel der Angstthemen. In: Koch, U. (Ed.): Sprachinhaltsanalyse in der psychosomatischen und psychiatrischen Forschung: Grundlagen- und Anwendungsstudien mit den Affektskalen von Gottschalk & Gleser. Beltz, Weinheim 1984 (im Druck).

Günther, U. und Groeben, N.: Abstraktheitssuffix-Verfahren: Vorschlag einer objektiven ökonomischen Messung der Abstraktheit/Konkretheit von Texten. In: Zeitschrift für experimentelle und Angewandte Psychologie 15(1): 55-74 (1978).

Guiter, H. and Arapov, M.V. (Ed.): Studies on Zipf's Law. Studienverlag Dr. N. Brockmeyer, Bochum 1982.

Haag, W.: Dokumentation von Anwendungssystemen aus der Sicht der Benutzer. Informatik und Operations Research, Schriftenreihe Band 9. S.Toeche-Mittler-Verlag, Darmstadt 1981.

Hedberg, B. and Mumford, E.: The Design of Computer Systems: Man's Vision of man as an Integral Part of the System Design Process. In: Mumford, E. and Sackman, H. (Eds.): Human Choice and Computers: 31-59, North-Holland, Amsterdam 1975.

Held, G., Stonebraker, M.R. und Wong, E.: INGRES: A Realtional Database System. Proc. Nat. Computer Conf. (Anaheim, Calif. May. 19-22): 409-416 (1975).

Henken, V.J.: Banality Reinvestigated: A Computer-Based Content Analysis of Suicidal and Forced Death Documents. Suicide 6(1): 36-43 (1976)

Henne, H. und Rehbock, H.: Einführung in die Gesprächsanalyse. Sammlung Göschen, de Gruyter, Berlin 1979.

Hennig, J. und Huth, L.: Kommunikation als Problem der Linguistik. Vandenhoeck & Ruprecht, Göttingen 1975.

Herczeg, M.: DYNAFORM - Ein interaktives Formularsystem zum Aufbau und zur Bearbeitung von Datenbasen. In: Balzert, H. (Hg.): Software-Ergonomie. German Chapter of the ACM Berichte Bd. 14: 135-146,Teubner, Stuttgart 1983.

Heß, K., Brustkern, J. und Lenders, W.: Maschinenlesbare deutsche Wörterbücher. Dokumentation, Vergleich, Integration. Niemeyer, Tübingen 1983.

Hörmann, H.: Meinen und Verstehen - Grundzüge einer psychologischen Semantik. Suhrkamp, Frankfurt 1976.

Hoffmann, K. und Poller, H.: Untersuchungen zum Selektionsprozeß in psychoanalytischen Behandlungsprotokollen. Med. Diss. Universität Ulm 1978.

IBM Corpo.: HIPO - A design aid and documentation technique. 1974,

Ince, D.C.: A Software Tool for Top-down Programming. Software-Practice and Experience 13: 687-695 (1983).

Inhetveen, R. und Luft, A.L.: Abstraktion, Idealisierung und Modellierung bei der Spezifikation, Konstruktion und Verifikation von Software-Systemen. Angewandte Informatik 12: 541-548 (1983).

Jackson, M.: System Development. Prentice-Hall, Englewood Cliffs 1983.

Jacob, R.J.: Using Formal Specifications in the Design of a Human-Computer Interface. Communications of the ACM 26(4): 259-264 (1983).

Jappe, G.: Über Wort und Sprache in der Psychoanalyse. Fischer, Frankfurt 1971.

Jochum, F.: Semantik-orientiertes Retrieval natürlichsprachlicher Texte. In: Wossidlo, P.R. (Hg.): Textverarbeitung und Informatik. Informatik-Fachberichte 30: 114-126, Springer, Berlin 1980.

Jochum, F. und Winter, E.: ISAC - Eine Analyse- und Entwurfsmethode für komplexe Softwaresysteme. Veröffentlichung Nr. 81/2 der Firma ACTIS, Stuttgart 1981.

Kächele, H.: Maschinelle Inhaltsanalyse in der psychoanalytischen Prozeßforschung. Unveröffentlichte med. Habil., Ulm 1976.

Kächele, H.: Zur Bedeutung der Krankengeschichte in der klinisch-psychoanalytischen Forschung. Jahrbuch für Psychoanalyse XII: 118-178 (1981).

Kächele, H.: Verbal Acitivity Level of Therapists in Initial Interviews and Long-Term Psychoanalysis. In: Minsel, W.R. und Herff, W. (Eds.): Methodology in Psychotherapy Research. Proceedings of the 1st European Conference on Psychotherapy Research. Trier 1981, Vol.1: 125-129, Lang, Frankfurt 1983.

Kächele, H.: Computer-Aided Analysis of Psychotherapeutic Discourse. - An Introduction to the Workshop. In: Minsel, W.R. und Herff W. (Eds.): Methodology in Psychotherapy Research. Proceedings of the 1st European Conference on Psychotherapy Research. Trier 1981, Vol. 1: 116-118, Lang, Frankfurt 1983.

Kächele, H., Grünzig, H-J. und Thomä, H.: Zur Urteilsbildung im psychoanalytischen Prozeß. Die Bedeutung des linear-additiven Modells. Medizinische Psychologie 5: 66-80 (1979)

Kächele, H., Hohage, R. und Mergenthaler, E.: Therapieorientierte Dokumentation in einer psychotherapeutischen Ambulanz - Funktion und Implikation. Psychotherapie, Psychosomatik, Medizinische Psychologie 33(4): 142-146 (1983).

Kächele, H. und Mergenthaler, E.: A Survey of Literature Refering to the Analysis of Data in Psychotherapy. In: Minsel, W.R. und Herff, W. (Eds.): Methodology in Psychotherapy Research. Proceedings of the 1st European Conference on Psychotherapy Research, Trier 1981, Vol. 1: 153-161, Lang, Frankfurt 1983.

Kächele, H. und Mergenthaler, E.: Auf dem Wege zur computerunterstützten Textanalyse in der psychotherapeutischen Prozeßforschung.

In: Baumann, U. (Hg.): Psychotherapie: Makro-/Mikroperspektive. Verlag für Psychologie, Dr. C.J. Hogrefe, Göttingen 1984.

Kächele, H., Schaumburg, C. und Thomä, H.: Verbatimprotokolle als Mittel in der psychotherapeutischen Verlaufsforschung. Psyche 10: 902-927 (1973).

Kächele, H., Thomä, H. und Schaumburg, C.: Veränderungen des Sprachinhaltes in einem psychoanalytischen Prozeß. Schweizer Archiv für Neurologie, Neurochirurgie und Psychiatrie 116: 197-228 (1975).

Kallmeyer, W. und Schütze, F.: Konversationsanalyse. Studium Linguistik 1: 1-28 (1976).

Katz, J.J. and Fodor, J.A.: The Structure of a Semantic Theory. In: Fodor, J.A. and Katz, J.J. (Eds.): The Structure of Language. Prentice-Hall, Englewood Cliffs 1964.

Keenan, E.L.: On Semantically Based Grammar. Linguistic Inquiry III(4): 1972.

Keutgen, H.: Rapid Prototyping. Informatik Spektrum 5(2): 125, (1982).

Klann-Delius, G.: Zur Transkription der Daten. Arbeitspapier Universität Bielefeld 1981.

Knauel, H.: Zauberwort "Textbank". Börsenblatt 18: 529-533 (1982).

Koberg, D. and Bagnall, J.: The UNIVERSAL TRAVELER - A Soft-Systems guide to: Creativity, Problem-Solving, and the Process of Reaching Goals. Kaufmann, Los Altos 1976. In Deutsch erschienen: Der Universal Reiseführer. Ein zuverlässiger Begleiter für alle, die Probleme lösen und Ziele erreichen wollen. Bauwelt, Berlin 1976.

Koch, U. (Hg.): Sprachinhaltsanalyse in der psychosomatischen und psychiatrischen Forschung: Grundlagen- und Anwendungsstudien mit den Affektskalen von Gottschalk & Gleser. Beltz, Weinheim 1984.

Köhler, R.: Modelle und Methoden der quantitativen Linguistik und ihr Verhältnis zur Inhaltsanalyse. Vortrag auf dem LDV-Kolloquium der Universität Trier 1983.

Köhler, R.: Zur Interpretation des Menzerathschen Gesetzes. In: NN. (Hg.): Glottometrika 6: Studienverlag Dr.N. Brockmeyer, Bochum 1984 (erscheint).

Köhler, R. und Altmann, G.: Semiotische Systeme. Zeitschrift für Semiotik V/4: (1983).

Kohut, H.: Introspektion, Empathie und Psychoanalyse. Suhrkamp-Taschenbuch, Frankfurt 1977.

Koolwijk, van J. und Wieken-Mayser, M.: Techniken der empirischen Sozialforschung. Oldenbourg, 1974 (Band 3).

Kops, M.: Auswahlverfahren in der Inhaltsanalyse. Hain, Meisenheim 1977.

Kowarski, I. and Michaux, C.: MIDOC: A Microcomputer System for the Management of Structured Documents. Information Processing 83: 567-572 (1983).

Krause, R.: Sprache und Affekt. Kohlhammer, Stuttgart 1981.

Krug, R. und Köhle, K.: Der Gebrauch von Personalpronomina als Indikator für Beziehungskonstellationen in Visitengesprächen. In: Köhle, K. und Raspe, H.H. (Eds.): Das Gespräch während der ärztlichen Visite: 178-195, Urban & Schwarzenberg, München 1982.

Kucera, H. and Francis, W.N.: Computational Analysis of Present-Day American English. Brown University Press, Boston 1967.

Küpfmüller, K.: Die Entropie der deutschen Sprache. Fernmeldetechnische Zeitschrift 7(6): 265-271 (1954).

Labov, W. and Fanshel, D.: Therapeutic Discourse - Psychotherapy as Conversation. Academic Press, New York 1977.

Lacan, J.: Fonction et champ de la Parole et du Langage en Psychoanalyse (1956): 237-322, Ecrits Senil, Paris 1966. In deutsch erschienen in: Haas, N. (Hg.): Schriften I: 73-169, Walter, Olten 1973.

Laffal, J.: An Approach to the Total Content Analysis of Speech in Psychotherapy. In: Shlien, J.M. (Ed.): Research in Psychotherapy: 277-294, American Psychological Association, Washington 1968.

Lang, H.: Die Sprache und das Unbewußte. Jaques Lacans Grundlegung der Psychoanalyse. Suhrkamp, Frankfurt 1973.

Lisch, R. und Kriz, J.: Grundlagen und Modelle der Inhaltsanalyse. Rowohlt (rororo) Hamburg 1978.

Lolas, F., Mergenthaler, E. and Von Rad, M.: Content Analysis of Verbal Behaviour in Psychotherapy Research: A Comparison between two methods. British Journal of Medical Psychology 55: 327-333 (1982).

Lorenz, M. and Cobb, S.: Language and a Woman's Place. Harper and Row, New York 1975.

Luborsky, L. und Spence, D.: Quantitative Research on Psychoanalytic Therpay. In: Garfield, S. and Bergin, A. (Eds.): Handbook of Psychotherapy and Behavior Change. Wiley, New York 1971 (2. Aufl. in: Bergin, A. and Garfield, S. (Eds.): 1978).

Lucas, H.C.: Why Information Systems fail. Columbia University Press, New York 1975.

Lüke, B.: Experimentelle Untersuchungen zum Benutzerverhalten in der Dialog-Finanzbuchhaltung. In: Balzert, H. (Hg.): Software-Ergonomie. German Chapter of the ACM Berichte Bd. 14: 288-300, Teubner, Stuttgart 1983.

Lundeberg, M., Goldkuhl, G. and Nilssen, A.: A Systematic Approach to Information Systems Development - I: Indroduction. Information Systems 4(1): 93-118 (1979).

Maddison, R.N. et al.: Information System Methodologies. In: Samet, P.A. (Ed.): BCS Monographs in Informatics. Wiley Heyden Ltd., Great Britain, 1983.

Mahl, G.F.: Disturbances and Silence in the Patient's Speech in Psychotherapy. Journal of Abnormal and Social Psychology 53: 1-15 (1956).

Mahl, G.F.: On the use of "ah" in Spontaneous Speech: Quantitative, Developmental, Characterological, Situational, and Linguistic Aspects. Amer. Psychol. 13: 349 (1958).

Mahl, G.F.: Measures of two Expressive Aspects of a Patient's Speech in two Psychotherapeutic Interviews. In: Gottschalk, L.A. (Ed.): Comparative Psycholinguistic Analysis of two Psychotherapeutic Interviews: 91-114, Int. Univ. Press, New York 1961.

Mahl, G.F.: Body Movement, Ideation, and Verbalization During Psychoanalysis. In: Freedman, N. and Stanley G. (Eds.): Communicative Structures and Psychic Structures: 291-310, Plenum Press, New York 1977.

Mergenthaler, E.: Bemerkungen zur computerunterstützten Sprachinhaltsanalyse. Vortrag 2. Werkstatt für Forschung in der Psychoanalyse, Ulm 1979.

Mergenthaler, E.: Das Textkorpus in der psychoanalytischen Forschung. In: Bergenholtz, H. und Schäder, B. (Hg.): Empirische Textwissenschaft. Aufbau und Auswertung von Text-Corpora. Scriptor-Verlag, Königstein/-Ts., 1979.

Mergenthaler, E.: Das Psychotherapie-Textarchiv in Ulm. Zentralarchiv für empirische Sozialforschung. Information 9. Köln 1981.

Mergenthaler, E.: Some Hints on Textual Data. Classifying, Archiving and Analyzing. In: Minsel, W.R. und Herff, W. (Eds.): Methodology in Psychotherapy Research. Proceedings of the 1st European Conference on Psychotherapy Research. Trier 1981, Vol. 1: 118-124, Lang, Frankfurt 1983.

Mergenthaler, E.: Die Transkription von Gesprächen. Eine Zusammenstellung der Regeln. Arbeitspapier Abteilung für Psychotherapie, Universität Ulm 1984. Auch erschienen in: ZUMA-Arbeitsbericht 84/01: 5-25, Mannheim 1984. (Teil 1)

Mergenthaler, E.: TEXT BASE MANAGEMENT Systeme - Werkzeuge zur Archivierung und Analyse sprachlicher Daten. Angewandte Informatik 6: 262-267 (1983).
Auch erschienen in: ZUMA-Arbeitsbericht 84/01: 56-64, Mannheim 1984. (Teil 2)

Mergenthaler, E. und Büscher, U: Benutzerhandbuch für das Programmsystem EVA zur automatisierten Inhaltsanalyse. Arbeitspapier Abteilung für Psychotherapie, Universität Ulm 1979.

Mergenthaler, E., Drewek, B. und Kemmer, U.: Benutzerhandbuch für das Textbanksystem. SFB 129, Universität Ulm, in Vorbereitung.

Mergenthaler, E. und Hössle, I.: Das Patientendokumentationssystem PADOS. Abteilung Psychotherapie, Ulm, in Vorbereitung.

Mergenthaler, E., Nafe, B. und Traue, H.: Zur prozeduralen Berechnung von Interaktionskennwerten. Arbeitspapier SFB 129, Universität Ulm 1984.

Mergenthaler, E. und Stöcklein, U.: FKON51: Ein Fortran-Konstruktor zur Datenerfassung am SIG51. Arbeitspapier Abteilung Psychotherapie, Ulm 1979.

Merten, K.: Inhaltsanalyse. Westdeutscher Verlag, Köln 1983.

Meyer, A.-E.: Psychoanalytische Prozeßforschung zwischen der Skylla der "Verkürzung" und der Charybdis der "systematisch akustischen Lücke". Zeitschrift Psychosomatische Medizin 27: 103-116 (1981).

Mills, H.D.: Mathematical Foundations for Structured Programming. IBM Document, Gaithersburg 1972.

MINDOK. Ein Informationssystem auf Kleinrechnern zur Erfassung, Verwaltung und Retrieval von Dokumenten und Daten. (Ausgabe 2.0) INFODAS GmbH, Köln 1983

Minsel, W.-R.: Beziehungen zwischen dem Erfolg von Psychotherapie und Sprachmerkmalen der Psychotherapeuten sowie ihrer Klienten. In: Nickel, G. (Hg.): Kongreßberichte der 2. Jahrestagung der Gesellschaft für Angewandte Linguistik: 157-161 (1971).

Mochmann, E. (Hg.): Computerstrategien für die Kommunikationsanalyse. Campus, Frankfurt 1980.

Mohler, P.Ph. und Züll, C.: TEXTPACK V-Kurzbeschreibung. ZUMA-Arbeitsbericht 84/01: 63-91, Mannheim 1984. (Teil 1)

Moles, A.A.: Informationstheorie und ästhetische Wahrnehmung. M.DuMont, Schauberg, Köln 1971.

Moritz, H.: Umsetzung wahrnehmungspsychologischer Erkenntnisse für die Informationsgestaltung am Bildschirm (Maskengestaltung). In: Balzert, H. (Hg.): Software-Ergonomie. German Chapter of the ACM Berichte Bd. 14: 98-113, Teubner, Stuttgart 1983.

Moser, U.: Affektsignal und aggressives Verhalten. Zwei verbal formulierte Modelle der Aggression. In: Psyche: Bd. XXXII: 229-258, 1978.

Moser, U.: Beiträge zu einer psychoanalytischen Theorie der Affekte. Berichte aus der interdisziplinären Konfliktforschungsstelle am Soziologischen Institut der Universität Zürich Nr. 10, Teil 1 (1983).

Moser, U., von Zeppelin, I. und Schneider, W.: Wunsch, Selbst, Objektbeziehung: Entwurf eines Regulierungsmodells kognitiv-affektiver Prozesse. Berichte aus der Interdisziplinären Konfliktforschungsstelle Nr. 9 vom Soziologischen Institut der Universität Zürich 1981.

Nake, F.: Schnittstelle Mensch-Maschine. In: Michel, K.M. und Spengler, T. (Hg.): Kursbuch 75. Computerkultur: 109-118, Rotbuch, Berlin 1984.

Nassi, I. and Shneiderman, B.: Flowchart Techniques for Structured Programming. SIGPLAN Notices: 13-26 (1973).

Neudert, L., Kübler, Ch. und Schors, R.: Die inhaltsanalytische Erfassung von Leiden im psychotherapeutischen Prozeß. In: Czogalik, D., Ehlers, W. und Teufel, R. (Hg.): Perspektiven der Psychotherapieforschung: Einzelfall-Gruppe-Institution. Hochschulverlag Freiburg 1984. (im Druck)

Norman, D.A.: Design Rules Based on Analyses of Human Error. Communications of the ACM 26(4): 254-258 (1983).

O'Dell, J. and Winder, P.: Evaluation of a Content-Analysis System for

Therapeutic Interviews. Journal of Clinical Psychology 31(4): 737-744 (1975).

Olle, T.W., Sol., H.G. and Verijn-Stuart, A.A. (Eds.): Information Systems Design Methodologies: A Comparative Review. Proceedings of the IFIP TC 8 Working Conference on Comparative Review of Information Systems Design Methodologies, Noordwijkerhout, The Netherlands, 10-14 May 1982. North-Holland, Amsterdam 1982.

Olle, T.W., Sol, J.G. and Tully, C.J. (Eds.): Information Systems Design Methodologies: A Feature Analysis. Proceedings of the IFIP WG 8.1 Working Conference on Feature Analysis of Information Systems Design Methodologies, York, UK, 5-7 July 1983. North-Holland, Amsterdam 1983.

Parunak Dyke Van, H.: Data Base Design for Biblical Texts. In: Bailey, R.W. (Ed.): Computing in the Humanities: 149-161, North-Holland 1982.

Paulus, W.: Planung und Entwicklung eines Programmsystems zur EDV-gestützten qualitativen Analyse von Verbaldaten. Vortrag auf dem ZUMA-Workshop: Datenmanagement bei qualitativen Erhebungsverfahren 1983. ZUMA-Arbeitsbericht 84/01: 65-90, Mannheim 1984. (Teil 2)

Pepinsky, H.B.: A Computer-Assisted Language Analysis System (CALAS) and its Applications. ERIC Document Reproduction Service, Arlington 1979.

Piller, E.: Der Einfluß der Rechnerarchitektur auf die Software-Ergonomie. In: Balzert, H. (Hg.): Software-Ergonomie. German Chapter of the ACM Berichte Bd. 14: 215-226, Teubner, Stuttgart 1983.

Ramsey, H., Atwood, M.E. and Doren van, J.R.: Flowcharts Versus Program Design Languages: An Experimental Comparison. Communications of the ACM 26(6): 445-449 (1983).

Reynes, R.: Lexical Differences between Working and Resistance Sessions in Psychoanalytic Psychotherapy. Journal of Clinical Psychology 1984 (in Press).

Rödiger, K.-H. und Nullmeier, E.: Arbeitswissenschaftliche und psychologische Kriterien für die Softwaregestaltung - was bleibt von den Ansprüchen und wie könnte man sie erfüllen? In: Balzert, H. (Hg.): Software-Ergonomie. German Chapter of the ACM Berichte Bd. 14: 278-287, Teubner, Stuttgart 1983.

Roome, W.D.: Programmer's Workbench: New Tools for Software Development. Bell.Lab.Rec. 57(1): 19-25 (1979).

Ross. D.T.: Structured analysis (SA) - a language for communicating ideas. IEEE Transactions on Software Engineering 1(3): 6-15 (1977).

Ruberg, W.: Untersuchung sprachlicher Reaktionen von Patienten auf Tonbandaufnahmen psychoanalytischer Behandlungen. Med. Diss. Universität Ulm 1981.

Ruoff, A.: Grundlagen und Methoden der Untersuchung gesprochener Sprache. Niemeyer, Tübingen 1973.

Ruoff, A.: Häufigkeitswörterbuch gesprochener Sprache. Niemeyer, Tübingen 1981.

Ryska, N. und Herda, S.: Kryptographische Verfahren in der Datenverarbeitung. Springer, Berlin 1980.

SALEM: Ein Verfahren zur automatischen Lemmatisierung deutscher Texte. Niemeyer, Tübingen 1980.

Sandig, B.: Zur Differenzierung gebrauchssprachlicher Textsorten im Deutschen. In: E. Gülich, E. und Raible, W. (Hg.): Textsorten: Differenzierungskriterien aus linguistischer Sicht. Frankfurt 1972.

Schank, R.C.: Language and Memory. Cognitive Science 4: 243-284 (1980).

Schaumburg, C.: Personalpronomina als Indikatoren interpersonaler Beziehungen. Rer. biol. hum. Diss., Universität Ulm 1980.

Schek, H.J. and Lum, V.: Complex Data Objects: Text, Voice, Images: Can DBMS Manage Them? Proceedings Ninth International Conference on Very Large Data Bases, Florence 1983.

Schlörer, J.: Probleme des Datenschutzes und der Datensicherung bei "anonymen" Daten. Med. Welt 29(19): 777-781 (1978).

Schmucker, B.: Entwurf und Implementierung eines Systems zur On-line-Transkription psychotherapeutischer Texte. Dipl.-Arbeit, Universität Ulm/Heidelberg 1981.

Schneider, H.-J. (Hg.): Lexikon der Informatik und Datenverarbeitung. Oldenbourg, München 1983.

Schöfer, G.: Das Gottschalk-Gleser-Verfahren: Eine Sprachinhaltsanalyse zur Erfassung und Quantifizierung von aggressiven und ängstlichen Affekten. Zeitschrift für Psychosomatische Medizin und Psychoanalyse 23: 86-102 (1977).

Schöfer, G.: Versuch der Anwendung der Gottschalk-Gleser-Sprachinhaltsanalyse auf Psychotherapiematerial. Therapiewoche 26(7): 1049-1057 (1976a).

Schöfer, G.: Erfassung affektiver Veränderungen durch Sprachinhaltsanalyse im Psychotherapieverlauf. Bibl. Psychiat. 154: 55-61 (1976b).

Schöfer, G.: Das Gottschalk-Gleser-Verfahren: Eine Sprachinhaltsanalyse zur Erfassung und Quantifizierung von aggressiven und ängstlichen Affekten. Zeitschrift für Psychosomatische Medizin und Psychoanalyse 23: 86-102 (1977).

Schott, G.: Automatische Deflexion deutscher Wörter unter Verwendung eines Minimal-Wörterbuchs. Sprache und Datenverarbeitung (SDV) 1: 62-77 (1978).

Schulz, A.: Vom CAD zum CAS: Angewandte Informatik 12: 607-614 (1982).

Schulz, A.: Methoden des Softwareentwurfs und Strukturierte Programmierung. Gruyter, Berlin 1982.

Schupp, J.: Möglichkeiten EDV-gestützter Strukturierung und Ordnung des qualitativen Interviews. ZUMA-Arbeitsbericht 84/01: 93-119 Mannheim 1984 (Teil 1).

Schwartz, A.: Toward a Computer Content Analysis of Concreteness. Undergraduate Psychology Major's Honor Thesis, University of New York 1980.

Sneed, H.: Programmentwurfs-Methoden im Vergleich. Online-adl-Nachrichten 9: 716-721 (1979).

SOFTECH Inc.: SADT. Structured analysis and design technique of SofTech, Inc. 1978.

Spence, D.P.: The Processing of Meaning in Psychotherapy: Some Links with Psycholinguistics and Information Theory. Behavioral Science 13(5): 349-361 (1968).

STAIRS. Dokumentationssystem zur Informationsspeicherung und -wiedergewinnung. IBM Deutschland GmbH, Bonn 1972.

Stelck, K.: SONIS. Social Network Investigation System. European Political Data Newsletter 50: 40-50 (1984).

Stone, P.J., Dunphy, D.C., Smith, M.S., and Ogilvie, M.: The General Inquirer: A Computer Approach to Content Analysis. The MIT-Press, London 1966.

Stonebraker, M., Stettner, H., Lynn, N., Kalash, J. and Guttman, A.: Document Processing in a Relational Database System. ACM Transactions on Office Information Systems 1(2): 143-152 (1983).

Stonebraker, M., Wong, E., Kreps, P. and Held, G.: The Design and Implementation of INGRES. ACM Trans. Database Syst. 1(3): 189-222 (1976).

Tausch, R.: Gesprächspsychotherapie. Hogrefe, Göttingen 1973.

Tausworthe, R.C.: Standardized Development of Computer Software. Part I Methods. Prentice-Hall, Inc., Englewood Cliffs, New Jersey 1977.

Teller, V. and Dahl, H.: Framework for a Model of Psychoanalytic Inference. Proceedings IJCA. 394-400, Vancouver 1981.

Thaller, M.: Datenbankorientierte Verfahren bei der maschinenunterstützten Auswertung historischen Quellenmaterials. In: Kneser, T. (Hg.): Datenverarbeitung in den Geisteswissenschaften, Göttingen 1980a.

Thaller, M.: Automation on Parnassus. CLIO - A Databank Oriented System for Historians. In: Historical Social Research / Historische Sozialforschung 15: 1980b.

Thaller, M.: CLIO: Ein datenbankorientiertes Programmsystem für Historiker. Manual Teil 1, Göttingen 1982.

Thaller, M.: CLIO: Ein datenbankorientiertes Programmsystem für Historiker. Manual Teil 2, Göttingen 1983a.

Thaller, M.: CLIO: Einführung und Systemüberblick. Manual, Göttingen 1983b.

Thaller, M.: Recycling the Drudgery. On the Integration of Software Supporting Secondary Analysis of Machine-Readable Texts in a DBMS. Computers in Literary and Linguistic Research. Proceedings of the VII International Symposium of the ALLC, Pisa 1982. Auch in: Linguistica Computationale III (83c) Supplement: 253-268 (1983c).

Thaller, M.: Ungefähre Exaktheit. Theoretische Grundlagen und praktische Möglichkeiten einer Formulierung historischer Quellen als Produkte 'unscharfer' Systeme. Max-Planck-Institut Göttingen, 1984a.

Thaller, M.: Ungenauigkeit und Effizienz. Die Informationsstruktur historischen Quellenmaterials und ihre Bearbeitung mit dem datenbankorientierten Programmsystem CLIO. Vortrag auf dem ZUMA-Workshop Datenmanagement bei qualitativen Erhebungsverfahren 1983. In: ZUMA-Arbeitsbericht 84/01. Datenbanksysteme für das Management sprachlicher Daten. Teil 2: 91-122 (1984b).

Thomä, H., Kächele, H. und Schaumburg, C.: Modell zur klinisch-empirischen Verlaufsforschung. Bericht, DFG-Projekt 170, Teil B, Ulm 1973.

Thomä, H. und Rosenkötter, L.: Audiovisuelle Hilfsmittel in der psychotherapeutischen Ausbildung. Didacta Medica 4: 108-112 (1970).

Thomä, H.: Schriften zur Praxis der Psychoanalyse: Vom spiegelnden zum aktiven Psychoanalytiker. Suhrkamp, Frankfurt 1981.

Toglia, M.P. and Battig, W.F.: Handbook of Semantic Word Norms. Wiley, New York 1978.

Traue, H.: Der Einsatz maschineller Inhaltsanalyse zur Untersuchung verbaler Interaktionen. In: Mackensen, R. und Sagebiel, F.: Soziologische Analysen, TUB-Dokumentation, Berlin 1979.

Verheijen, G.M.A. and Van Bekkum, J.: NIAM: An Information Analysis Method. In: Olle, T.W., Sol, H.G. and Verijn-Stuart, A.A. (Eds.): Information Systems Design Methodologies: A Comparative Review. Proceedings of the IFIP TC 8 Working Conference on Comparative Review of Information Systems Design Methodologies, Noordwijkerhout, The Netherlands. North-Holland, Amsterdam 1982.

Wallerstein, R. und Sampson, H.: Issues in Research in the Psychoanlytic process. Int. J. Psychoanal. 52: 11-50 (1971).

Walther, E.: Abriß der Semiotik. Arch +2, H. 8: 3-13 (1969).

Wedekind, H.: Systemanalyse - Die Entwicklung von Anwendungssystemen für Datenverarbeitungsanlagen. Hanser, München 1973.

Weinrich, H.: Großer Mann - was nun? Die Zeit 3: (1975).

Weizenbaum, J.: Die Naturwissenschaft und der zwanghafte Programmierer. Psyche 3: 268-285 (1976). Original in: Weizenbaum, J.: Computer Power and Human Reason. From Judgment to Calculation. W.E. Freemann, San Francisco 1976.

Weizenbaum, J.: Die Macht der Computer und die Ohnmacht der Vernunft. Suhrkamp, Frankfurt 1977.

Westmeyer, H.: Wissenschaftstheoretische Grundlagen der Einzelfallanalyse. In: Petermann, F. und Heht, F.J. (Hg.): Fortschritte der Klinischen Psychologie 18, Einzelfallanalyse: 17-34, Urban und Schwarzenberg, München 1979.

Willee, G.: LEMMA - Ein Programmsystem zur automatischen Lemmatisierung deutscher Wortformen. Sprache und Datenverarbeitung. Bd. 1/2, 3. Jahrg:

45-60 (1979).

Willee, G.: Das Programmsystem LEMMA 2 - Eine Weiterentwicklung von 'LEMMA'. IKP-Arbeitsberichte Nr. 2. Universität Bonn 1982.

Willee, G.: Möglichkeiten einer maschinellen Auswertung der Texte von Jargon-Aphatikern. GAL-Vortrag, Heidelberg 1984.

Winkler, P.: Notationen des Sprechausdrucks. Zeitschrift für Semiotik 1: 211-224 (1979).

Winkler, P.: Markierungen paraphonetischer Information: Kurventypen, Kombinationen und Strukturen. In: Köhler, R. and Boy, J.: Glottometrika 5: 168-202, Studienverlag Dr. N. Brockmeyer, Bochum 1983.

Winograd, T.: Understanding Natural Language. Academic Press, New York 1972.

Wirth, N.: Program Development by Stepwise Refinement. Communications of the ACM 14(4): 221-227 (1971).

Wirtz, E.M. and Kächele, H.: Emotive Aspects of Therapeutic Language: A Pilot Study on Verb-Adjective-Ratio. In: Minsel, W.R. and Herff, W. (Eds.): Methodology in Psychotherapy Research. Proceedings of the 1st European Conference on Psychotherapy Research. Trier 1981, Vol.1: 130-135, Lang, Frankfurt 1983.

Wodak, R.: How do I put my Problem? Problem Presentation Therapy and Interview. Text 1:2(11): 191-213 (1981).

Wright, P. and Lickorish, A.: Proof-Reading Texts on Screen and Paper. Behaviour and Information Technology 2(3): 227-235 (1983).

Zadeh, L.A.: Fuzzy Sets. Information and Control 8: 338-353 (1965).

Zadeh, L.A.: Coping with the Imprecision of the Real World. Communications of the ACM 27(4): 304-311 (1984).

Zemanek, H.: Elementare Informationstheorie: 47-61, Oldenbourg, München 1959.

Zeppelin von, I.: Skizze eines Prozeßmodells der Psychoanalytischen Therapie. Psychologisches Institut der Universität Zürich 1981.

Zimbardo, Ph.G., Mahl, G.F. and Barnard, J.W.: The measurement of speech disturbance in anxious children. Journal of Speech and Hearing Disorders 28(4): 362-370 (1963)

Zimmer, J.M. and Cowles, K.H.: Content Analysis using FORTRAN. Journal of Counseling Psychology 19(2): 161-166 (1972).

Appendix A

The Transcription of Conversational Exchanges

A Summary of the Rules

CONTENTS

Introduction

The following rules for the transcription of conversational exchanges were chosen to suit the following requirements:

1. Good legibility of the transcribed material
2. As little effort as possible in the transcription
3. Computertolerability of the transcript.

It was only possible to meet these demands by makes compromises. This point is particularly relevant to the possible use of transcripts in scientific investigations. The rules were developed with reference to the kind of questions asked in scientific research into linguistic material provided by psychotherapeutic sessions. Specific linguistic problems (e.g. intonational phenomena) cannot be investigated using this procedure.

Reasons of research economy made it necessary to create a corpus of rules which would enable typists to produce high-quality transcripts in a single step and (possibly) also proofread it in a second step. As scientific personnel are scarce, this is an important point of consideration.

Computer tolerability, finally, was to guarantee that further processing of transcripts does not create excessive software problems. "Score notation", for example, which is commonly used in some places, was therefore not included. It is possible, however, to convert the recorded data into a "score". This is done with the help of special printing programs.

The ULM TEXTBANK receives a great proportion of its texts from institutions outside Ulm which are without computers. It was for this reason that a procedure for the transformation of data into a computer processable form was included in the rules. Moreover, due to recent technological progress, it is possible to carry out on-line transcriptions on microcomputers, providing the necessary support is given (e.g. in the correction of typing mistakes). In the future this development will be given greater impetus. The ULM TEXTBANK is planning to install mobile units for the recording of texts.

A General Remarks

All sounds audible on the tape recording are included in the transcript. These are: verbal, paraverbal, and nonverbal utterances of the speakers involved, and noises occurring in the situational context.

1. **Verbal utterances**
   These are all words which were spoken as whole words or parts of words. They are reproduced in "literary script", which orients itself on the spelling of written language, but considers only those sounds which are heard. Dialect forms are transcribed in their corresponding standard language forms (but cf. rule B 4). German examples:

   is, hab, habs, ne, gschafft

2. **Paraverbal utterances**
   These are all sounds or sound sequences which usually appear alone, not as part of complete sentence structures. These sounds often serve as conversational gap fillers, expressing feelings of doubt, confirmation,insecurity, thoughtfulness, etc. They are treated like sentences and are also recorded in literary script. Examples:

   hm, eh, ui, s, f

3. **Nonverbal utterances**
   These are all other noise-producing actions of the speaker. They are recorded where they occur in the form of comments.

   (coughs loudly), (laughs), (sighs)

4. **Noises occurring in the situational context**
   These are produced by the environment and are part of the communicative situation. They are recorded in the form of short comments. Examples:

   (telephone rings), (aeroplane passing)

B Symbolization of Particular Conversational Features

Special symbols are introduced for the indication of particular conversational features. These symbols are inserted in the text in order to emphasize particular parts of speech to mark quotations and indicate changes in the way of speaking. A further group of symbols (punctuation marks) is used in order to mark speech rhythm. The following examples will illustrate in detail how these symbols should be used:

1. **Emphasis and lengthening of sounds**
   Words which are clearly emphasized by the speaker are followed in the in the transcript by an exclamation mark. Where a sound is noticeably lengthened, a colon is entered behind it. A text sample with one lengthened and one emphasized sound looks as follows:

   well: if you do that!

2. **Names**
   Personal names, town names, and geographical names are replaced with pseudonyms (marked with a preceding asterisk). Within a given text pseudonyms ought to be used consistently.

   yesterday *Paul said, that Mr *McIntosh

3. **Quotations**
   Direct speech and quotations are distinguished from other contributions of the speaker by single question marks. Example:

   then he shouted 'leave me alone' or something

4. **Changes in way of speaking**
   If a speaker changes his way of speaking and says a few words in a voice that differs from his usual way of speaking, these words are enclosed in double quotation marks and transcribed in literary script. The variant may be characterized in a subsequent comment. German example:

   dieses ewige "Gschnader" (Swabian) haengt mir

5. **Punctuation**

Punctuation marks are inserted to mark rhythmic or syntactic caesures än the course of speech. They are chosen with regard to the height of intonation. Parts of speech enclosed in punctuation marks are called "cadences". The following marks are used:

? ascending cadence / cadence ending on a high note
= hovering cadence / cadence ending on a middle note
, descending cadence / cadence ending on a fairly deep note
. cadence ending on the key note
; unfinished cadence

Therefore the meaning symbols '.' and ',' correspond largely with their usage in written language. The symbol '?', on the other hand is used differently. It is here employed exclusively in indicating a raising of the voice. This usage differs from its usage in written language as marking a question.

Punctuation marks are inserted whenever a cadence is apparent, i.e., where the speaker pauses or changes the height of intonation (gradually or suddenly).

Punctuation marks are inserted immediately after the relevant word. In the following text example the speaker begins a sentence with "you said", but then starts again with "you know":

no= no. or yes? you said; you know

6 **Simultaneity**

Where two speakers are talking at the same time, this is also indicated in the transcript. With a view to computer-aided analysis, simultaneous passages must be transcribed one after the other. A plus sign preceding the first speaker's utterance marks the onset of simultaneity. One continues with the transcription of this speaker's contribution until the end of simultaneity is reached. The change in speaker is noted down and the other speaker's contribution transcribed up to the point where simultaneity ends, whereupon another plus sign is inserted. If the second speaker carries on talking, the transcription continues without a change in speaker. Otherwise one continues with the first speaker's contribution after recording the simultaneous passages. In cases where only parts of words are spoken simultaneously, whole words are transcribed as occurring simultaneously. In the following example "A/" and"P/" are used to distinguish the two speakers:

P/ I am suffering from +phlebitis
A/ yes= yes.+ said so before this

7. **Incomplete words**
   A hyphen immediately precedes or follows a word which was broken off either by the speaker himself or by a partner who has interrupted him. Text example:

   yest- I have the feeling, that

8. **Indistinguishable utterances**
   For every indistinguisable word an oblique is entered in the transcript. If more than one word is indistinguishable, the number of obliques should correspond with the number of the words the transcriber could not understand. The obliques are seperated by spaces. Text example:

   there I have / / / as it / be

   Alternatively one can amend the text by entering the suspected wording in double brackets. Example:

   yesterday ((morning)) I did

9. **Pauses**
   Pauses are indicated by one hyphen or a sequence of hyphens. The number of hyphens depends on the length of the pause and can be inferred from the following table:

duration of pause	number of hyphens		increase/hyphen
2 sec	1	-	2 sec
5 sec	2	--	3 sec
10 sec	3	---	5 sec
15 sec	4	----	5 sec
start using stopwatch at this point			
30 sec	5	-----	15 sec
1 min	6	------	30 sec
2 min	7	-------	1 min
5 min	8	--------	3 min
10 min	9	---------	5 min
15 min	10	----------	5 min
30 min	11	-----------	15 min
more	12	------------	

As is apparent in the table, pauses of less then 2 seconds are not recorded. The following procedure is recommended for the estimation of pauses: Up to 15 seconds, increases should be discriminated by counting (e.g. "21, 22, 23" for 3 seconds). A stop watch should be used to measure the length of longer pauses.

It must be emphasized, that the next hyphen must not be entered until the time limit is reached, i.e. verbal exchange was not resumed for the full period of time which alone warrants another hyphen. Text example:

I don't know, --- today

Pauses are to be attributed always to the speaker who was speaking last. This goes particularly for silences which are broken by another speaker.

10. **Time elapse**
Information concerning the time that has elapsed since the beginning of the exchange is given in the form of a comment in brackets. A subsequent apostrophe indicates minutes, two apostrophes indicate seconds. Example:

(+3'10")

11. **Interjections**
In spoken language interjections usually represent independent cadences. Their various different meanings can be recorded with the help of punctuation marks. The following table listing the

variants of the particle "hm" should serve as an example:

usage		meaning
hm	hmhm	confirmation
hm?		question
hm=	hmhm=	hesitation
hm,	hmhm,	astonishment
hm.	hmhm.	helplessness

12. **Ambiguity**
With a view to computer-aided analysis, it may be advisable to convert ambiguous utterances into unambiguous ones. It is possible to enter any number of alternative wordforms or figures behind an oblique. A figure can represent the number of a word's possible meanings. In the case of pronouns it is possible to name their antecedents behind the oblique. The basis vocabulary can serve as a tool in the search for the possible meanings of a word. Examples:

match/2, we/group, there/Ulm

13. **Commentary**
Apart from the standard comments mentioned above, other (free) comments may be made. These should be enclosed in parentheses, which have not been taken up by any of the rules above.

14. **Division of words at the end of a line**
A word is divided (at the end of a line) by a subsequent Ö% sign. One carries on with the second part of the word on the next line. The division need not follow the rules of syllabification in this case. Text example:

the shop closing tim%
es have been changed.

15. **Discontinuous forms**
This rule refers to the notation of composite nouns, which occur frequently in the German language. In spoken German, the root which is common to two word forms with different prefixes or suffixes is omitted from one word and the two word forms are linked with a conjunction. In this case one indicates the omission by attaching a dash. This rule also applies to the omission of pre-

fixes and suffixes, where they are shared by two words. Two German examples:

An- und Abflug, Hauptfrage und -antwort
(arrival and departure of flight, main question and answer)

16. **Omissions**
The apostrophes customary in written language are not employed in transcriptions. Instead a new word form is created in accordance with the principles of literary script. Examples:

Its raining now, Id rather go now

17. **Umlauts and "ß"**
The so-called "sharp s" or "ß" is transribed as "s$". Umlauts are transcribed as "a$", "o$", and "u$" respectively. German examples:

ich weis$, das$ bei scho$n Wetter

18. **Use of small or capital initial letter**
All words except nouns and personal names begin with a small letter. The same goes for the beginning of sentences.

19. **Abbreviations**
In spoken as opposed to written language, abbreviations do not exist. Accordingly, words which usually take an abbreviated form are spelled out (as they are spoken). Example:

for example (instead of 'e.g.')

20. **Stuttering**

Stuttered words are treated like incomplete words, i.e., the stuttered word particles are followed by a hyphen and a space. This procedure is repeated once for every time this particle can be heard. Text example:

I ha- ha- have not done it

21. **Numbers, fractions, etc.**
    Figures, fractions are written out in full where possible. Only typical figures are transcribed as such. Examples:

    eleven, two thirds, 1981, James Bond 007, firstly

22. **Neologisms**
    Words tied together to form new words are transcribed with the help of hyphens. German examples:

    das In-der-Welt-Sein, schwarz-weis$

23. **Mistakes**
    Slips of the tongue and other mistakes are transcribed as fully as possible. German examples:

    allergerisch, Definieres eh Definiertes
    (instead of 'allergisch' resp. instead of 'Definiertes')

24. **General points**
    Where several rules apply, only one should be applied to guarantee legibility of the transcript.
    Spelling should follow DUDEN (the standard spelling dictionary of the German language) or its equivalent like Webster's New Collegiate Dictionary.

C Transcription Standard

The transcription of conversational exchanges should generally be carried out in three distinct stages during which all the rules listed in par A and B should be applied.

The **first** stage contains the actual process of transcription. A "raw transcript" is produced by putting the data on computer-readable file or alternatively, by feeding them into the microcomputer system TELECOMP on-line. Rules B10 and B12 are neglected at this stage. This first version of the transcript then goes through the admission module of the textbank system, which generates a provisional draft and prints it in its modified form.

In a **second** step this draft of the transcript is compared with the original recording. Necessary alterations (changes and corrections) are made by hand. The complete exchange is then listened to again and rule B10 is applied (i.e., time elapse is marked in 5-minute intervals). A correction program finally deals with alterations and time data within the textbank itself.

The **third** step concerns the application of rule B12. A second draft has been generated automatically by the textbank system and contains the assigned antecedents and alternative meanings. The codings may be checked (and altered if necessary) at the terminal with the help of an interactive program.

The transcript thus passes through three stages. The following table below lists the different levels of transcriptional status.

Level	**Description**
0	other rules or only some of them were observed.
1	all rules were strictly observed except rules B10 (time elapse) and B12 (ambiguities).
2	all rules except B12 (ambiguities) were strictly observed.
3	all rules were observed.
V	during the transcription not all rules were observed. An accompanying note contains information about the rules, which were not applied.

A record card is kept for every conversational exchange that is being transcribed in order to keep track of the standard reached by a transcript. The card contains information regarding the following items: Name of transcriber, duration of transcription, date of transcription, level of transcript, name of corrector, duration of correction, date of correction, level of correction, and length of conversational exchange.

For technical aspects concerning the layout of machine readable documents please contact the ULM TEXTBANK. A copy of the actual rules and technical guidelines will be provided for you .

Appendix B

Tables

size of probe ALFA=0.01

p(%)	Nmin	p(%)	Nmin
0.01	52980	0.51	1036
0.02	26488	0.52	1016
0.03	17658	0.53	997
0.04	13243	0.54	978
0.05	10593	0.55	960
0.06	8827	0.56	943
0.07	7566	0.57	926
0.08	6620	0.58	910
0.09	5884	0.59	895
0.10	5295	0.60	880
0.11	4814	0.61	865
0.12	4412	0.62	851
0.13	4072	0.63	838
0.14	3781	0.64	825
0.15	3529	0.65	812
0.16	3308	0.66	800
0.17	3114	0.67	788
0.18	2940	0.68	776
0.19	2785	0.69	765
0.20	2646	0.70	754
0.21	2520	0.71	743
0.22	2405	0.72	733
0.23	2300	0.73	723
0.24	2204	0.74	713
0.25	2116	0.75	703
0.26	2035	0.76	694
0.27	1959	0.77	685
0.28	1889	0.78	676
0.29	1824	0.79	668
0.30	1763	0.80	659
0.31	1706	0.81	651
0.32	1653	0.82	643
0.33	1602	0.83	635
0.34	1555	0.84	628
0.35	1511	0.85	620
0.36	1469	0.86	613
0.37	1429	0.87	606
0.38	1391	0.88	599
0.39	1355	0.89	592
0.40	1321	0.90	586
0.41	1289	0.91	579
0.42	1258	0.92	573
0.43	1229	0.93	567
0.44	1201	0.94	560
0.45	1174	0.95	555
0.46	1149	0.96	549
0.47	1124	0.97	543
0.48	1101	0.98	537
0.49	1078	0.99	532
0.50	1057	1.00	527
p(%)	Nmin	p(%)	Nmin

size of probe ALFA=0.05

p(%)	Nmin	p(%)	Nmin
0.01	36886	0.51	721
0.02	18442	0.52	707
0.03	12294	0.53	694
0.04	9220	0.54	681
0.05	7375	0.55	668
0.06	6146	0.56	656
0.07	5267	0.57	645
0.08	4609	0.58	634
0.09	4096	0.59	623
0.10	3687	0.60	612
0.11	3351	0.61	602
0.12	3072	0.62	593
0.13	2835	0.63	583
0.14	2633	0.64	574
0.15	2457	0.65	565
0.16	2303	0.66	557
0.17	2168	0.67	548
0.18	2047	0.68	540
0.19	1939	0.69	532
0.20	1842	0.70	525
0.21	1754	0.71	517
0.22	1674	0.72	510
0.23	1602	0.73	503
0.24	1535	0.74	496
0.25	1473	0.75	490
0.26	1416	0.76	483
0.27	1364	0.77	477
0.28	1315	0.78	471
0.29	1270	0.79	465
0.30	1227	0.80	459
0.31	1188	0.81	453
0.32	1150	0.82	448
0.33	1115	0.83	442
0.34	1083	0.84	437
0.35	1052	0.85	432
0.36	1022	0.86	427
0.37	995	0.87	422
0.38	968	0.88	417
0.39	944	0.89	412
0.40	920	0.90	408
0.41	897	0.91	403
0.42	876	0.92	399
0.43	856	0.93	394
0.44	836	0.94	390
0.45	817	0.95	386
0.46	800	0.96	382
0.47	783	0.97	378
0.48	766	0.98	374
0.49	750	0.99	370
0.50	735	1.00	367
p(%)	Nmin	p(%)	Nmin

size of probe ALFA=0.01

p(%)	Nmin	p(%)	Nmin
0.1	5295	5.1	101
0.2	2646	5.2	99
0.3	1763	5.3	97
0.4	1321	5.4	95
0.5	1057	5.5	93
0.6	880	5.6	91
0.7	754	5.7	90
0.8	659	5.8	88
0.9	586	5.9	87
1.0	527	6.0	85
1.1	479	6.1	84
1.2	438	6.2	82
1.3	404	6.3	81
1.4	375	6.4	80
1.5	350	6.5	78
1.6	328	6.6	77
1.7	309	6.7	76
1.8	291	6.8	75
1.9	276	6.9	74
2.0	262	7.0	73
2.1	249	7.1	71
2.2	238	7.2	70
2.3	227	7.3	69
2.4	218	7.4	68
2.5	209	7.5	67
2.6	201	7.6	67
2.7	193	7.7	66
2.8	186	7.8	65
2.9	180	7.9	64
3.0	173	8.0	63
3.1	168	8.1	62
3.2	162	8.2	61
3.3	157	8.3	61
3.4	153	8.4	60
3.5	148	8.5	59
3.6	144	8.6	58
3.7	140	8.7	58
3.8	136	8.8	57
3.9	133	8.9	56
4.0	129	9.0	56
4.1	126	9.1	55
4.2	123	9.2	54
4.3	120	9.3	54
4.4	117	9.4	53
4.5	115	9.5	53
4.6	112	9.6	52
4.7	110	9.7	51
4.8	107	9.8	51
4.9	105	9.9	50
5.0	103	10.0	50
p(%)	Nmin	p(%)	Nmin

size of probe ALFA=0.05

p(%)	Nmin	p(%)	Nmin
0.1	3687	5.1	70
0.2	1842	5.2	69
0.3	1227	5.3	67
0.4	920	5.4	66
0.5	735	5.5	65
0.6	612	5.6	64
0.7	525	5.7	62
0.8	459	5.8	61
0.9	408	5.9	60
1.0	367	6.0	59
1.1	333	6.1	58
1.2	305	6.2	57
1.3	281	6.3	56
1.4	261	6.4	55
1.5	244	6.5	54
1.6	228	6.6	54
1.7	215	6.7	53
1.8	203	6.8	52
1.9	192	6.9	51
2.0	182	7.0	50
2.1	173	7.1	50
2.2	165	7.2	49
2.3	158	7.3	48
2.4	151	7.4	47
2.5	145	7.5	47
2.6	140	7.6	46
2.7	134	7.7	46
2.8	129	7.8	45
2.9	125	7.9	44
3.0	121	8.0	44
3.1	117	8.1	43
3.2	113	8.2	43
3.3	109	8.3	42
3.4	106	8.4	42
3.5	103	8.5	41
3.6	100	8.6	41
3.7	97	8.7	40
3.8	95	8.8	40
3.9	92	8.9	39
4.0	90	9.0	39
4.1	88	9.1	38
4.2	85	9.2	38
4.3	83	9.3	37
4.4	81	9.4	37
4.5	80	9.5	36
4.6	78	9.6	36
4.7	76	9.7	36
4.8	74	9.8	35
4.9	73	9.9	35
5.0	71	10.0	35
p(%)	Nmin	p(%)	Nmin

Author Index

Lecture Notes in Medical Informatics

Vol. 23: Selected Topics in Image Science. Edited by O. Nalcioglu and Z.-H. Cho. IX, 308 pages. 1984.

Vol. 24: Medical Informatics Europe 1984. Proceedings, 1984. Edited by F. H. Roger, J. L. Willems, R. O'Moore and B. Barber. XXVII, 778 pages. 1984.

Vol. 25: Medical Informatics Europe 1985. Edited by F. H. Roger, P. Grönroos, R. Tervo-Pellikka and R. O'Moore. XVII, 823 pages. 1985.

Vol. 26: Methodical Problems in Early Detection Programmes. Proceedings, 1983. Edited by E. Walter and A. Neiß. XIII, 198 pages. 1985.

Vol. 27: E. Mergenthaler, Textbank Systems. VI, 177 pages. 1985.

GPSR Compliance
The European Union's (EU) General Product Safety Regulation (GPSR) is a set of rules that requires consumer products to be safe and our obligations to ensure this.

If you have any concerns about our products, you can contact us on

ProductSafety@springernature.com

In case Publisher is established outside the EU, the EU authorized representative is:

Springer Nature Customer Service Center GmbH
Europaplatz 3
69115 Heidelberg, Germany

www.ingramcontent.com/pod-product-compliance
Ingram Content Group UK Ltd.
Pitfield, Milton Keynes, MK11 3LW, UK
UKHW051450290926
15471UKWH00008B/1116
* 9 7 8 3 6 6 2 1 0 3 0 1 2 *